Do All Bugs Need Drugs?

Conventional and Herbal Treatments of Common Ailments

Deborah Hodgson-Ruetz

iUniverse, Inc.
New York   Bloomington

Do All Bugs Need Drugs?
Conventional and Herbal Treatments of Common Ailments

iUniverse books may be ordered through booksellers or by contacting:

iUniverse
1663 Liberty Drive
Bloomington, IN 47403
www.iuniverse.com
1-800-Authors (1-800-288-4677)

Because of the dynamic nature of the Internet, any Web addresses or links contained in this book may have changed since publication and may no longer be valid.

ISBN: 978-1-4502-6826-4 (sc)
ISBN: 978-1-4502-6828-8 (dj)
ISBN: 978-1-4502-6827-1 (ebk)

Printed in the United States of America

iUniverse rev. date: 1/3/2011

Contents

Author's Note vii

Introduction ix

Part 1: Congestion 1

Chapter 1: Colds and Flu 3

Chapter 2: Sinus Congestion. 13

Chapter 3: Lung Congestion. 19

Chapter 4: Liver Congestion. 23

Part 2: Stomach Problems 27

Chapter 5: Heartburn 29

Chapter 6: Constipation 33

Part 3: Reproductive Organ Problems 39

Chapter 7: Yeast Infection 41

Chapter 8: Premenstrual Syndrome. .47

Chapter 9: Menstrual Cramps. 53

Chapter 10: Heavy Menstruation (Menorrhagia) 59

Chapter 11: Menopause 63

Chapter 12: Hysterectomy 69

Chapter 13: Prostate Health 71

Part 4: Pregnancy 77

Chapter 14: Early Pregnancy. 79

Chapter 15: Late Pregnancy 85

Part 5: Life and Lifestyle: **95**

Chapter 16: Eyestrain 97

Chapter 17: Depression. 101

Chapter 18: Chronic Fatigue Syndrome 109

Appendix 1: Glossary 115

Appendix 2: Tonics and Formulas .123

Appendix 3: Capsule Explanation .127

Appendix 4: Some Essential Vitamins 129

Appendix 5: References. 131

Author's Note

This book is intended as a reference book only, not as a medical guide or manual for self-treatment. If you suspect that you have a serious medical problem, please seek competent medical care. The information here is designed to help you make informed choices about your health. It is not intended as a substitute for any treatment prescribed by your doctor. The information about herbal remedies and treatments is intended to increase your knowledge about the latest developments in the use of plants for medical purposes. Because every individual's body is unique, however, a physician must diagnose conditions and supervise the use of healing herbs to treat individual health problems. Herbs and other natural remedies are not a substitute for professional medical care. I urge you to seek out the best medical resources available to help you make informed choices.

In this book I have only touched on a few of the more common problems today, in a hope that it will bring relief to a few of those who try them. I believe God gave all plants to all the people; we need to share this knowledge of plants as medicines in order to save plants and ourselves. The study of herbs and their medicinal properties is becoming a lost art. I think it would be a great tragedy to keep this knowledge a secret, because when healing plants become extinct, and the people who use them, then the medicine is lost and the secret is useless. I only hope that this book will inspire interest in the study of herbs. Some herbs have been exploited by commercialization as fad herbs. A caution is needed, do not take herbs without studying the benefits and dangers of them first.

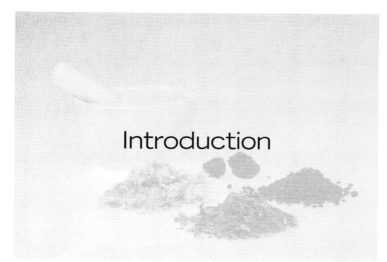

Introduction

Some of the more dramatic, chronic health problems facing modern populations can be easily cured by natural substances. So many of the ailments we suffer can be related to lifestyles and diet. The immune system, for example, is the focus of tremendous scientific interest because of its relation to diseases such as cancer, leukemia, chronic fatigue syndrome, AIDS, and severe allergies. Yet the immune system is weakened by pharmaceuticals. In contrast, the immune system is strengthened by herbs, such as echinacea, astragalus, and reishi.

Hippocrates may be the father of medicine, but for centuries medieval Europe followed the teachings of Galen, a second-century physician, who wrote extensively about the body's four "humors"— Blood, phlegm, black bile, and yellow bile—and classified herbs by their essential qualities as hot or cold, dry or damp. These theories were later expanded by seventh-century Arabian doctors. This medicine is practiced today in the Muslim world and in India.

It is difficult to determine when plants were first used as a healing medium and how prehistoric peoples discovered specific uses for plants. It has been established through written records in the Middle East and China thousands of years ago, that discovery was through intuition, experimentation and food usage.

Ayurvedic, one of the oldest known forms of medicine, claims to have been presented by the gods from the beginning of time. In Europe use of botanicals goes back to the beginning of recorded history. To this day, herbalists in European clinics conduct some of the best research on plant use.

In America early settlers brought their folklore from Europe, adding this to the abundant knowledge of the Native American Indians. The Indians have many tales of how the Great Spirit gave certain medicinal plants for the use of the people.

The basic ideas of the philosophy regarding the human body as being controlled by a "vital force" are an active part of homeopathic philosophy today.

We have a long and proven history of restoring health to the people of the world. We are proving the old ways with solid science. With the knowledge we are gathering today from the labs herbalists will again have a respected place among healers. Our aim is not to treat the surface symptoms but to treat underlying conditions that influence the whole organism. Herbalists assist the body's tendency to move toward internal harmony.

Billions of dollars are spent on medical and hospital care. Most of this goes to surgery, synthetic drugs, and doctors' fees. Some people are now realizing that it is far better to spend reasonable amounts of money on good nutrition and natural remedies. The public purse cannot afford the expensive and expanding hospital system, especially as the average age of people increases. Almost as important in healing people, herbs are natural and grow in our backyard. Herbs can and will bring down the cost of health care and bring the nation to health. Herbology is now stepping forward as a complementary form of medicine for a modern world.

Part 1:
Congestion

Chapter 1:
Colds and Flu

I am sure that none of us need a description of what a cold or flu is like. It's easy to recall the brain-mashing headache, the major muscle aches, the bone-tired fatigue, the vomiting, and the fever that makes you sweat and shiver. These are all clues that the flu has its hold on you.

Anyone who has had the flu before will probably be tempted to get the flu shot before the season begins, and a shot can prevent the flu or lessen its severity. But if it strikes, most of the recovery action is on the home front. The flu shot only works on *the* flu virus that it is designed to prevent. There are millions of flu viruses in the air, and if you're exposed to a flu virus, it is quite possible that the shot you received did not immunize you from that particular virus.

The ancient Greeks thought leech-induced bleeding was the answer to a cold or the flu. More recently, mom's answer was her chicken soup. And guess what? While we still spend more than one billion dollars each year on cold remedies—nothing to sneeze at—we have yet to find a single way to make the common cold less common.

The good news is that the older you get, the less likely you are to fall victim to any of the two hundred different viruses that cause a cold. Children typically get six to ten colds a year, because their immune systems haven't matured; adults usually get two to four colds annually. While scientists are currently working on high-tech ways to stop cold viruses from spreading, it's best to avoid the cold in the first place. An ounce of prevention is worth a pound of cure in this case.

Conventional Treatments for Colds and Flu

Drink vitamin C-rich juice. Orange, tomato, grapefruit, or pineapple juice can help you get over cold. But you need to drink about five glasses a day, according to Dr. Jahre Jeffrey, a clinical associate professor of medicine at Temple University. Studies have shown that it takes a lot of vitamin C (about two thousand milligrams) to reduce sneezes and coughs in cold sufferers. This is supported by the respiratory research lab at the University of Wisconsin.[1] If that amount seems like a bit much to swallow, you can take vitamin C supplements. But don't go overboard; larger doses of vitamin C can cause stomach upset in some people.

Consuming any hot liquid helps to cut through congestion, but chicken soup is probably the best of all. No study has shown why chicken soup seems to work so well, but it is certain that the tasty soup is a comforting way to get protein and other nutrients if you are not up to eating. It seems that people who wouldn't drink hot water will readily sit down to a cup of chicken soup.

Keep a glass of water on your nightstand. Taking sips of water during the night is another way to moisten the sinuses and help breathing. It also helps combat the dehydration that can result from fighting colds.

Pump your legs; a daily 45 minute walk can help speed recovery from colds. A daily walk helps shake up and spread out the natural killer cells—the Marine Corps of your immune system—making them more vigilant. But don't push yourself. Exhaustive exercise can actually impair the immune system. If you pace yourself so that you can comfortably talk while you walk, you're going at the right speed.

Don't bother with antihistamines. Over-the-counter cold medicines that contain antihistamines do little more than make you sleepy. Findings have proven that histamine is not produced when you have a cold, so the drug designed to fight it won't help. Antihistamines may stop your runny nose, but they may also do more harm than good. "Antihistamines dry up mucous membranes, which are already irritated," says Dr. David N. Gilbert, director of the Chiles Research Institute and the department of medical education at the Providence Medical Centre, Portland, Oregon. "They thicken the nasal mucus

---

1   Renner, John, and the Consumer Health Information Research Institute. 1993. *The Home Remedies Handbook by the Editors of Consumer Guide and Hundreds of Leading Doctors.* Louis Weber Publications Int., Lincolnwood, IL, p. 89.

so you feel like you need more decongestant, and they can cause an irritated cough."[2]

To treat headaches, be selective. Studies have shown that aspirin and acetaminophen (the active ingredient in Tylenol) actually increase nasal blockage and reduce the level of virus-fighting antibodies. If you have a headache, ibuprofen may be the better choice. If your child has a headache along with a cold, ask your pharmacist for a dosage of ibuprofen that is suitable for a child. Never give a child aspirin without consulting a doctor, because it can contribute to Reye's syndrome, a life-threatening neurological condition.

For a stuffy nose, nasal sprays are safer and more effective than oral decongestants. If you use them for longer than three days, however, your nose will become stuffier than ever. So after you have used a nasal spray for a couple of days, switch to a commercial saline solution, or make one yourself. Dissolve a teaspoon of salt in a pint of water, and then use a nose dropper to drop it in your nose. Gently blow your nose on a tissue.

If you have a cold, sit in a sauna. There is no sure way to prevent a cold, but the Swedes may be on the right track. If you indulge in a sauna twice a week or more, you are less likely to catch a cold. It is possible that the high temperatures may block cold viruses from reproducing in your body, and that by sweating, the body eliminates toxins within it. The humidity also helps with the cleansing of the mucus membranes. A healthy house is a clean house. A healthy body is clean inside and out. So having a sauna is like cleaning your house.

Make your home tropical. It is not the cold weather but the lack of humidity that is the major issue in catching colds. Overheated homes and offices are the perfect setup for a cold. When our noses and tonsils are dry, they cannot trap germs efficiently. It becomes difficult to sneeze and cough, so it's difficult to expel germs from the body. Turning down the thermostat and turning on a room humidifier keeps viruses-laden mucus flowing out of your body.

In a study involving more than four hundred people, researchers at Carnegie Mellon University in Pittsburgh and Britain's common cold unit found that participants who reported high levels of psychological

---

2 Renner, John, and the Consumer Health Information Research Institute. 1993. *The Home Remedies Handbook by the Editors of Consumer Guide and Hundreds of Leading Doctors.* Louis Weber Publications Int., Lincolnwood, IL, p. 89.

stress were twice as likely to develop a cold as those reporting low stress levels. This study is a first step in understanding a complex issue. Whether diminishing daily stress has an actual impact on your likelihood to get a cold is unknown, but it just may help defend you against a season of sniffles.

When it comes to the flu, you need vitamins and minerals to mount an effective defense against the bug. Aim for well-balanced meals. If you don't have much appetite, try to have something healthy and comforting, like some bland fruit, such as mashed bananas or applesauce.

Drinking your nutrients is a good idea when you have the flu especially if you're not up to eating solid foods. Wash down your meals with a vitamin-rich juice such as vegetable juice, or have a bowl or two of soup. The more fluid you drink, the more your tissues are hydrated, and the more readily mucus flows out of your body.

Combination cold/flu liquid remedies can contain *as much as* 80 proof alcohol. Most of the flu medications that had high alcohol content have been taken off the market. Other flu medications that have a high alcohol content now have to be purchased through the pharmacist or doctor, because that equals to the amount in a shot of liquor. Alcohol can depress your immune system and also dry out your mucous membranes, so you should avoid it when you have the flu.

Toss your old toothbrush. Cold and flu viruses continue to linger on wet toothbrush bristles, and you can reinfect yourself day after day. To prevent this, throw away your toothbrush three days after the onset of the flu and use a new one.

Steer clear of crowds. The greater your exposure too many people, the more likely you are to have contact with a cold or flu virus. Spending time in offices, malls, theaters, or other crowded environments between December and February increases your chances of ending up flat on your back with the flu, especially if your resistance is low.

Avoid flying in airplanes if you can. There was a flu outbreak in Atlanta many years ago, and the local office of the Centers for Disease Control traced an outbreak of flu to a single infected passenger in an airplane. Due to a faulty ventilation system, the air inside the cabin recirculated the flu virus as the plane sat waiting for takeoff. Later, thirty-eight of the fifty-four people on the flight came down with the flu. There have not been follow up studies, but an airplane has cramped quarters and air blowing all around, which may create a high-risk situation. There is no way to get fresh air into the cabin of an airplane. So they recirculate the old air and add oxygen to it.

Ordinary soap kills the flu virus, but in order to reduce your chances of infection, you have got to remember to wash your hands throughout the day, not just before meals or after going to the bathroom. When a family member is sick, frequently use a disinfectant spray on the sink and countertops. Use hot, soapy water to wash towels, telephones, and dishes. Just by using good cleaning techniques (using soap and water) you can get rid of 89 percent of most germs and viruses. Carry a hand sanitizer with you when you go out. Many hand sanitizers come in convenient purse- or pocket-size now. Some restaurants even have hand sanitizers at the entrance. In Canada and Mexico especially, I have seen many restaurants using hand sanitizers at the entrance. This is ever increasing with the spread of the new super viruses in 2009 and 2010.

Humidify a room to help lick the flu. The vapor emitted by a room humidifier moistens the mucous membranes in your nose and throat, so germs are more easily trapped and expelled. If you use an ultrasonic room humidifier, be sure to rinse it out daily to prevent mold and fungus growth in the water reservoir. You should also run a hot water and bleach mixture through the machine at least once a week, following the directions on the humidifier. Better yet, use a hot steam humidifier that moisturizes and kills any microbial growth in the water.

Relaxation techniques may protect you from influenza and other infections, but you don't have to engage in self-hypnosis to get the benefits of relaxation therapy. Other ways to relax include deep breathing and stretching, meditation, and yoga.

Like many maladies, a little exercise can make a big difference in your healing. Pump your legs—a daily forty-five-minute walk can help speed recovery from colds. A daily walk helps shake up and spread out the natural killer cells—the Marine Corps of your immune system—making them more vigilant. If you pace yourself so that you can comfortably talk while you walk, you're going at the right speed. But don't push yourself. If you have the flu (rather than a cold), you're probably better off avoiding exercise. Exhaustive exercise can actually impair the immune system and slow your recovery. After your symptoms clear (which usually takes about a week) wait another two weeks before returning to your regular exercise schedule.

Herbal Treatments for Colds and Flu

For general immunity problems, I strongly recommend cleansing the internal body with kombucha before you get sick. Kombucha, also known by some as Manchurian mushroom, is a fermented beverage with a real zing in it. I can personally attest to the attributes of this herb (actually it is living yeast). It is great. It tastes like apple juice, or if left to steep for a while, like apple cider vinegar. Use caution with kombucha, because too much can cause a healing crisis. A healing crisis feels like having the flu, with aches and pains, sweating, and the like. This can last for days (unlike the flu, which lasts for a week or two), until the body catches up to the flu virus and can start healing again.

Another way to strengthen the overall immune system is to try huang qi (*Astragalus membranaceus*). Huang qi increases the production of white blood cells and strengthens the immune response; it has antibacterial properties and as an energy tonic it strengthens Wei qi, or defense energy. It also reduces the toxicity in the liver. You take it as a decoction of tincture. For debilitated conditions, add other energy tonics, such as licorice, dang qui, and bai hu. Huang qi is not recommended if your condition involves excess heat or a yin deficiency.

A final recommendation for a generally weak immune system is purple coneflower (*echinacea spp.*). It is an antibacterial and antiviral agent; it strengthens resistance to infections and is useful for all septic or infectious conditions. Take five hundred milligrams powdered root in capsules or ten milliliters tinctures. Repeat up to four times a day. Use as simple, or add phlegm-reducing remedies like elderflower and catnip, or fever herbs like yarrow or boneset, depending on symptoms. In high doses, purple coneflower can cause occasional nausea and dizziness, so be prudent in your usage.

The remaining herbal-based recommendations are specifically for colds and flu. If you've got the chills, try a ginger tea made with a teaspoon of ground ginger in boiling water. The Chinese use a formula of five slices of ginger with slices of the white of five green onions, boiled in water for five minutes. This cold and flu remedy can be very beneficial and can serve as a semi diaphoretic (will increase perspiration) during the first stages of congestion.

Break up congestion with a bowl of chili or other spicy foods containing horseradish, hot pepper sauce, hot mustard, or curry—the hotter the better! Hot Mexican or Indian foods are good congestion busters: as a rule of thumb, if it makes your eyes water, it will make your nose run.

Garlic (*Allium sativum*) is an antimicrobial and antifungal; it's suitable for a wide range of infectious conditions. Eat up to six fresh cloves a day in acute conditions, or take commercial capsules. It is best as a simple herb, and you can diminish the odor by eating parsley. Note, however, that garlic may irritate your stomach. If it does, take ginger or fennel tea. Avoid therapeutic doses of garlic during pregnancy and lactation.

Gui zhi (*cassia*) warms cold conditions; promotes sweating; and is an antibacterial agent. Take as a decoction or tincture; use cinnamon bark, also known as rou GUI, if GUI zhi is unavailable. For chills, mix with a little fresh ginger root. Don't use these herbs if you're pregnant. Because it is also a potential uterine stimulant if used in therapeutic doses especially the essential oils. Use the herb with care in overheated or feverish conditions.

Boneset (*Eupatorium perfoliatum*) promotes sweating and reduces fever. It is also an expectorant and it's good for hot feverish colds and influenza with muscle pain. It is said to be a good immunostimulant, which increases resistance in viral infections. Take an infusion or tincture three to four times a day. For feverish colds and influenza, combine with yarrow, elderflower, and peppermint. In high doses, boneset can cause vomiting, so don't overdo it.

Catnip (*Nepeta cataria*): yes, cat nip for colds is not as wacky as it sounds. Your cat loves it and you will too. It cools fevers and promotes sweating; it is an astringent and helps in alleviating mucous congestion. Take an infusion or tincture three to four times a day for feverish colds. Catnip can be mixed with yarrow, elderflower, boneset, ground ivy, angelica, or mulberry leaf to enhance their specific uses, as noted above.

One remedy for persistent flus and colds, if you can get the patient to comply, is the wet sheet treatment. In this program, the person who is sick is first put into a bath that is as hot as comfortable. This bath is prepared with the addition of two ounces of mustard and two ounces of ginger. While the patient is in the bath, he is given as much yarrow tea as he can drink. After about ten to fifteen minutes, the person is helped out of the bath and immediately wrapped in a cotton sheet that has been soaked in ice cold water. (As an alternative, you can put a wet sheet in the freezer.) The patient, wrapped in the cold sheet, is then wrapped in another sheet (this one dry), and then a wool blanket. He is left to sleep through the night. In the morning, when the person is unwrapped, he usually feels much better. The sheet is often covered with stains of the toxins that have come out overnight.

Goldenseal has been called the "king" of the mucous membranes and has gathered other honors as well. The Cherokee Indians introduced goldenseal as a medicine for the treatment of ulcers and arrow wounds. It has since gained a reputation as a very powerful herbal remedy. The root is bitter and unpleasant to taste but is very successful in treating stomach flu, slight food poisoning, and cold-swollen glands. A formula to use is:

3 parts goldenseal

1 part myrrh

1 part cayenne.

This formula and variations of it are quite famous as a cold/flu remedy. It is also good for general infections.

A formula is especially useful when the flu is associated with a headache is

4 parts goldenseal

1 part capsicum

1 part skullcap

When I was a child my mother always gave me chamomile tea. I do not know if she knew why it was good for me, but I always felt better when I had it. It is a diaphoretic that produces a good flow of blood to the body surface. It soothes and softens the skin, and increases the circulation to the stomach, nerves, and uterus. It is excellent for colds and fevers.

Prepared as an infusion, chamomile tea is soothing to the stomach. If a little ginger is added, it is good for colic, loss of appetite, and a sluggish intestinal canal. When preparing chamomile, the vessel should be kept covered to prevent steam from escaping. A lot of the medicinal properties are in the vapor. For a healing vapor bath, slowly simmer chamomile flower in a pot, cover your head with a towel, and breathe in the vapor. This is beneficial for colds, coughs, the flu, and lung problems.

Lastly, another good treatment for influenza is the peppermint formula, which appears in Appendix 2.

Chapter 2:
Sinus Congestion

It doesn't take much to get a stuffy nose. With every breath you take, you subject your nasal membranes to everyday irritants such as pollen, dust, cat dander, and particles of air pollution—all of which can clog things up faster than rush-hour traffic. In fact, just about any substance in the air can stuff a sensitive nose. And of course, you already know what a cold can do to block up your nasal passages. Did you know that you come in contact with about more than one hundred different cold germs daily?

Well, breathe easy—or at least easier, because there are plenty of ways to unblock that stuffiness. (Because nasal congestion and colds are often treated similarly, some of the information that follows is the same as that provided in connection with treating colds and flu.)

Sinusitis is an inflammation or infection of the sinus cavities in the skull. It often follows a cold but may be associated with dental problems, such as a deep-seated root abscess. It tends to affect tense people who do not express their emotions and who find it difficult (or are unwilling) to cry.

Key symptoms (as if I have to tell you how you felt the last time you were congested) are pain affecting sinus areas and headache (which may be severe). Sinuses may be tender to the touch and you may experience a nasal discharge often streaked with blood. Before the infection hits, you will feel pain radiating from your nose to the blocked sinus. If the sinuses remain clogged, you may develop a fever, a nasty taste in your mouth, or bad breath. Any of these symptoms may lead you to believe that you have a full-blown sinus infection.

Conventional Treatments for Sinus Congestion

Sniff an onion. Basically the only benefit you get from rubbing on menthol or other decongestants is some irritation that stimulates the nose to run and unblocks the stuffiness. You get the same effect from smelling an onion.

Go heavy on the spices. The cure for a stuffy nose is to make it runny, and few things make it run faster than a spicy meal. Eat some hot chili peppers; they will trigger a reflex response to make your nose runny.

Like when you have a cold, try some of Mom's chicken soup, or any other hot liquid taken from a cup. When you drink anything hot, the steam of the liquid helps unclog nasal passages, and the fluid itself helps dilute mucus in the nose and makes breathing easier. Besides soup, hot tea with lemon, and even hot water, are excellent decongestants

Hit the showers. Breathing the steam from a hot shower or bath is probably the easiest way to cut mucus and keep it from getting thick—a common cause of stuffiness.

A humidifier certainly helps put moisture in the air, but it can be counterproductive if it also spreads water impurities, spores, and germs. Use distilled water to fill humidifiers and you won't be filling your room with impurities. Clean the unit weekly by circulating a solution of half water, half white vinegar. The solution should be run through the unit for ten to fifteen minutes near an open window to avoid the creation of a vinegar odor. Then discard the vinegar solution and fill the unit with fresh distilled water. The unit can run for up to a week without cleaning again. Keeping open pans of water near the stove and radiators can also help to humidify a room, but the water needs to be changed frequently.

Use decongestant spray sparingly. You should use it no more than twice a day for a minimum of three or four days in a row. After that, take an equal amount of time off the medication, particularly when the relief it provides begins to wane, or when you notice that its effectiveness lasts for a shorter time. If that happens, there is a good chance that you are becoming dependent, and it is time to stop.

Over-the-counter decongestants are among the most potentially addictive of all drugs. Not only do many people get hooked on them, but the sprays can also damage the cells lining the nose. The sprays can cause the cells to lose their microscopic hairs, or cilia, which are crucial for keeping the normal mucous coating in the nose moving. It is difficult to wean yourself from nasal sprays, because the resulting congestion is so bad. "Advertisements touting relief from sinus pressure, congestion and pain are everywhere. Do they deliver what they promise? In the short run, nasal decongestants and nose drops may afford some relief," says Dr. Joel R. Saper, director, Michigan Headache and Neurological Institute, Ann Arbor, Michigan. "But if your sinuses are the problem, use for a long period of time puts you at risk for a chronic situation of diminishing returns." Because of the withdrawal from the constricting effects of the spray, you may experience more discomfort and more congestion as the medication wears off.

Unlike decongestant spray, nasal saline spray may be used indefinitely. With saline versions, you just moisten the membranes in your nose, which helps you breathe easier. And you don't need to buy the spray at a pharmacy; you can mix a batch of home brew by dissolving one-quarter teaspoon of table salt and one-quarter teaspoon of baking soda in about eight ounces of water. With a small atomizer or nose dropper, squirt one or two droppers of the solution up your nose as often as necessary. Saline soothes and cleans out things that are aggravating the congestion. It doesn't, however, provide extended relief or actually clear up the congestion.

Swallow some relief. Any of the over-the-counter oral decongestants usually are fine to take for a stuffy nose. But they should be used with caution by people with heart problems, high blood pressure, or urinary tract problems. They also interfere with other medication, especially antidepressants, so before you try any of them, ask your doctor or pharmacist first. Oral decongestants may aggravate an irregular heartbeat and can counteract medication to reduce high blood pressure. People who have urinary tract problems may find themselves having difficulty urinating if they take an oral decongestant.

Keep booze in the bottle. Substances in fermented alcoholic beverages can clog your nose as easily as they cloud your mind. Almost anyone who gets recurrent colds or sinus problems has congestion problems when he drinks alcohol.

When a newborn gets a stuffy nose, it can be particularly irritating—for both parent and child. Babies under three months are obligatory nose breathers, which simply mean they won't breathe through their mouths. So when a baby gets a stuffy nose, it's inordinately stressful. Many parents come rushing into the emergency room or pediatrician's office because their baby won't eat or sleep and is cranky all the time. It is because the baby's nose is stuffed up. A baby cannot suck on a bottle or feed if he can't breathe through his nose. To relieve an infant's stuffy nose, first use a bulb syringe or a nasal aspirator to clear the nose of as much mucus as you can. Then fill a medicine dropper with saline solution. Holding the baby in your arms, position him so that his head is slightly below the rest of his body and drop the saline into each nostril. You are doing it right if the saline hits the top of the baby's mouth. Immediately after spraying, hold the baby upright. Be sure to give one quick squirt in each nostril—so you don't flood the baby's nose with the saline and drown the child.

If your sinuses are congested, watch out for milk and wheat allergies. A number of people have an allergy to milk that is different from lactose intolerance: it congests the ducts in the nose. If that is causing your discomforts, you can see a fairly dramatic response with the elimination of milk products. Approximately 10 percent of sinus congestion sufferers feel enormously better when they stop consuming milk. Sensitivity to wheat may also cause congestion.

Zinc seems to have a specific effect on the nose. Zinc supplements have been used to treat people whose sense of smell has diminished, and zinc may improve congested sinuses as well. Take a fifty-milligram supplement daily, and continue to take the supplement if you notice an improvement.

Vitamin C has been advocated for the common cold, but it could spell relief for people with stuffed-up noses in general. Vitamin C in varying doses may bring relief, but you shouldn't take more than five hundred milligrams daily without a doctor's consent.

Another trick to help get rid of stuffiness is to raise the head of the bed. Lying on your back tends to build up the pressure of nasal fluid. Try raising your head by placing a few blocks or books under the bedposts, or sleeping on more than one pillow. Both help the nose drain. And don't lounge around in bed when you are congested; that gives mucus more chance to pool in your head rather than drain.

As with almost all maladies, work out to work it out. Exercise is a natural decongestant for common nasal stuffiness. When you walk, you stimulate better breathing and better blood circulation. Walking also helps shrink nasal membranes, and besides, you get a good breath of fresh air.

Herbal Treatments for Sinus Congestion

Like with a cold, the use of spices is a good remedy. As I said earlier, the cure to a runny nose is to make it runny. Few things make it run faster than a good bowl hot, hot chili. This running helps break up the congestion and remove irritants that may be causing the stuffiness.

The first herb of choice would probably be goldenseal, which is also in the clinical respiratory formula in Appendix 2. This formula is good for colds as well as sinusitis. Goldenseal is a powerful cooling astringent; it reduces phlegm. Take one four to five hundred milligrams in a capsule of powder or one milliliter tincture three times a day. Add eyebright powder to capsules. Avoid goldenseal if you are pregnant or if you have high blood pressure.

A good phlegm reducing herb is ground ivy (*Glechoma hederacea*). It is an astringent and has a drying effect on mucus in the sinuses and bronchi. Take as an infusion or tincture. It can be used with other phlegm-reducing herbs like elderflower or ribwort plantain. Use two parts ground ivy to one part other herb.

Bayberry is warming herb, and is an astringent; it stimulates the circulatory system. Use in powder form as a snuff, or add five milliliters of tincture to twenty milliliters emulsifying ointment and use as a sinus massage. For an antiseptic and antispasmodic effect, add two to three drops eucalyptus oil to the ointment. This herb should not be used in very hot conditions.

Cang er zi (*Xanthium sibiricum*) is a warming, phlegm-reducing agent. It is useful for sinus headaches and allergic rhinitis. Take this herb as a decoction or tincture. It is generally used in complex combinations, along with ten to fifteen other herbs, to produce specific actions. For sinusitis, add herbs like xin yi (Magnolia liliflora), lian qiao, or mulberry bark. Cang er zi can cause a dramatic fall in blood sugar if taken in high doses, so please be careful when using it.

A formula that is supposed to be effective for sinus problems is the horseradish formula. Combine one-third teaspoon fresh grated horseradish with one-third teaspoon apple cider vinegar. It should be chewed thoroughly with the mouth closed and then swallowed. This should be done three times per day, and the amount eaten should be increased by one-third teaspoon every three days until a full teaspoon is used. The procedure should be continued for one to four months even though the problem may appear to have been remedied. The vapor is very effective for inhibiting microorganisms. When the sinigrin and myrosin combine in the apple cider vinegar they create a volatile oil that goes up into the sinuses. The cleansing action of this formula is very irritating

Chapter 3:
Lung Congestion

There are many reasons why the lungs may be congested. The first thing to do is a through assessment of the patient. Check out to see if the congestion is due to an allergy or aspiration pneumonia (foreign body in the lungs). If it is due to bronchitis, you will hear wheezes in the chest when you listen to it. If it is due to pneumonia, you will hear a sound like water bubbling when you listen to the chest. If the chest sounds clear, the congestion may be in the upper airways. If there are no lung sounds when you listen to the chest, the lung may be collapsed, or there may be so much congestion that no air can get into it. In most cases, the patient's description of what it feels like when he breathes will help to diagnose the problem. You have to be careful not to confuse a heart condition with a chest cold—pleurisy feels a lot like a heart attack, but the pain is not as severe.

Bronchitis is inflammation of the bronchi, which may be due to infection. Chronic bronchitis is often exacerbated by common colds or associated with smoking and pollution. A key symptom of bronchitis is a productive cough, often with yellow phlegm. Bronchitis may produce the most nastiest-looking phlegm you have ever seen, but this aspect of the condition is arguably more unpleasant than a real cause for concern. It occurs because the mucus membranes lining the air passages in the chest become irritated and to soothe the irritation, the body makes secretions to coat the airways. This produces a build-up of gunk in the lungs, which must be cleared by coughing (and often a lot of sputtering, more than a '67 Chevy in dire need of a tune-up). In addition to the cough, bronchitis sufferers also often experience a raised temperature, chest pains, and breathlessness. Like the common cold, bronchitis affects nearly everyone at sometime in his life. Viruses cause temp increase and act fast. Acute cases are usually caused by a virus and will clear up on their own in a week or two, but with the new viruses coming out and SARS they are lasting longer. Chronic cases are just that. They last for years. And get worse as the years go on. Chronic cases, however, are almost always caused by smoking—either your own habit or long-term exposure to second hand smoke—and these cases may last for months. Chronic Bronchitis does not usually come with a high fever.

Conventional Treatments for Lung Congestion

Drink plenty of fluids to combat congestion. They help the mucus become more watery and easier to cough up. While warm liquids like mom's chicken soup may make you feel better, a cool glass of water, juice, or any other nonalcoholic beverage may work just as well. (All beverages are the same temperature in the body.) To avoid losing fluids from your body, doctors advise staying away from booze, because it can actually cause dehydration. Also avoid caffeinated products such as coffee, tea and cola because they make you urinate more and you may actually lose more fluids than you gain.

Get away from cigarettes. Even being near someone who smokes can make bronchitis worse or cause repeated episodes. You need to avoid all tobacco smoke. Even if you don't smoke but you are exposed to exhaled smoke, you are doing what is called passive smoking, and that can give you bronchitis.

If you do smoke, quitting is the most important thing you can do, since this habit has been linked to as much as 95 percent of all cases of chronic bronchitis. Your bronchitis will clear up when you quit smoking. Note that some new ex-smokers experience increased coughing and sputum production for a week or two after quitting. This is actually a good sign—the airways are sweeping out a lot of accumulated secretions. These symptoms usually subside after two to four weeks.

Even though a bronchial infection is not in the lung tissue itself, it is getting quite close to the lungs, which is always a worry for physicians. Because the bronchial passages are already irritated, the added inflammation resulting from a bronchial infection also makes medical attention more of a necessity for smokers or people who are affected by second hand smoke.

Plug in a vaporizer. If you have mucus that is thick and difficult to cough up, a vaporizer will help loosen the secretions. If you don't have a vaporizer, either run a hot shower with the bathroom door closed or fill the sink with hot water, put a towel over your head and the sink to create a tent, and inhale the steam for five to ten minutes every couple of hours. Don't rely on expectorants. Over-the-counter cough medicines may suppress your cough, which is the opposite of what you want. Besides, there is no evidence that they help dry up mucus. You will get better and cheaper results by drinking lots of liquids.

Bronchitis is usually not a serious problem, but you should see your doctor if: 1) your cough doesn't improve or worsens after one week (sometimes an X-ray is required to distinguish bronchitis from pneumonia), 2) you are coughing up blood, 3) you are elderly and get a hacking cough on top of another illness, 4) you are short of breath and have a very profuse cough, 5) you have asthma or another pulmonary condition that weakens your lungs and your ability to breathe easily, 6) you have a very high fever (over 101°F or 40°C) that lasts more than three days.

Herbal Treatments for Lung Congestion

In general, be aware that all herbs used to alleviate bronchitis are also good for the treatment of asthma.

Try elecampane (*Inula helenium*). It is a lung tonic and expectorant; it is restorative and warming and its food for weakened lungs and stubborn coughs. Take a decoction, tincture, or syrup. Use as a simple, or add ten milliliters of horsetail juice to heal lung damage; other restorative lung herbs that can be added include hyssop, white horehound, and anise.

White horehound (*Marrubium vulgare*) is an antispasmodic, a demulcent, and an expectorant. It relaxes the bronchi and eases congestion. Take as an infusion, tincture, or syrup, or suck horehound candy (which is available commercially). It can be combined with tonics like elecampane or hyssop, or warming expectorants like angelica. Use two parts white horehound to one part additional herb.

Cowslip (*Primula veris*) is a potent expectorant and is good for loosening old phlegm and easing stubborn, dry coughs. Take as a decoction, tincture, or syrup. Cowslip can be combined with strong expectorants like bloodroot and soothing demulcents such as ribwort plantain or licorice. Use two parts cowslip to one part additional herb. Do not take high doses of cowslip if you are pregnant, and avoid it if you're taking warfarin.

Thyme (*Thymus vulgaris*) is an antiseptic and expectorant. Thyme is useful for thick, infected phlegm and dry, difficult coughs. Take it as an infusion, tincture, or syrup. For a chest rub, mix ten drops essential oil in twenty milliliters of almond oil. You can add additional expectorants such as mulberry bark or healing herbs like horsetail for damaged lungs; the chest rub can be enhanced with five drops hyssop or peppermint essential oil. Thyme is another herb that should be avoided if you are pregnant. The clinical respiratory formula (in Appendix 2) is a formula that is well known. This formula is specific for dilating the bronchial tubes while cleansing the mucus from the chest. It has been found useful in airborne allergies, sinus congestion, and lung problems. Ma huang, the major ingredient of this herbal formula, has been a major part of Chinese medicine for over five thousand years. Its major chemical component, ephedrine (used extensively in western medicine since 1923), works on the autonomic nervous system to cause dilatation of the bronchial tubes and alveoli. It has also been shown to be a great cleaner of the respiratory mucous membranes.

Other herbs that are good for treating bronchitis include mullein leaves and coltsfoot leaves, which are expectorants, demulcents, and diuretics. As I mentioned earlier, goldenseal is considered the king of mucous membranes, building the quality while regulating the quantity. Lobelia herb works on the nerve supply to the lungs and is also an excellent expectorant. Cayenne stimulates blood circulation and supplies nutrients. It has been called the purest and most certain stimulant in the herbal materia medica.

Chapter 4:
Liver Congestion

In our polluted society, liver congestion is very common. It can manifest itself as a pathological disorder, but it often simply involves feelings of anger and stagnation. Key symptoms include a tendency for constipation; abdominal bloating; emotional irritability; menstrual disorders; red, itching palms, small red spots on the abdomen and sore, itching eyes.

Cirrhosis is a chronic disease of the liver that involves the destruction of liver cells. A common cause is excessive use of alcohol.

Jaundice is a symptom of liver problems. Jaundice occurs when there are excessive bile pigments circulating in the blood. It enters the mucous membranes and the skin, giving them the characteristic yellow pigmentation. Apart from the typical yellow appearance of the skin, jaundice generates such symptoms as body itching, vomiting with bile (indicated by the green appearance and bitter taste of vomit). Jaundice is also often accompanied by diarrhea with undigested fats present in the stools, and an enlargement of the liver, with pain and tenderness in the upper right quadrant of the abdomen.

Conventional Treatments for Liver Disease

Surgery may be necessary to remove the stones that may be in the bile duct or other obstructions. If there is bacterial infection in the liver, then antibiotic therapy is necessary. If you have jaundice and experience itching, use calamine lotion.

Herbal Treatments for Liver Disease

Milk thistle (*Cardus marianus*) encourages liver cell renewal and repair in degenerative conditions, such as when the liver has suffered from too much alcohol. Take as an infusion; or take up to ten milliliters tincture a day in hot water that has been allowed to cool down. Use as a simple herb, or add vervain, dandelion root, or globe artichoke and five drops goldenseal as additional liver tonics.

Bayberry bark's ability to heal the mucous membranes and to stimulate circulation has made it useful for cleaning out the liver and promoting glandular activity. An effective powder consists of the following components:

4 oz. bayberry bark powder

2 oz. ginger powder

1 oz. pinus spruce

1 tbsp. cloves powder

1 tbsp. cayenne pepper.

Mix the ingredients and then pass them through a fine sieve at least twice. Use one teaspoon of the formula to one cup of boiling water. Allow the infusion to steep, and then drink. If prepared in capsule form take two "0" capsules, three to four times a day.

Chai hu (*Bupleurum chinense*) is a bitter liver tonic; it encourages energy flow. Add ten grams of the herb to six hundred milliliters of water for a decoction. Combine with bai shao Yao, chuan xiong, goldenseal, and dandelion to help regulate liver function.

Gentian (*Gentiana lutea*) is a bitter, and a tonic, as well as a general digestive and liver stimulant. It has also been used for anorexia nervosa. Add fifteen grams root to six hundred milliliters of water for a decoction; take one to five drops tincture on the tongue per dose. Add tinctures of dandelion root, vervain, holy thistle, or barberry as additional liver tonics and stimulants, up to a combined total dose of five milliliters tincture

Dandelion root (*Taraxacum officinale*) is a very good root for a lot of things. It is a restorative tonic for liver functions; it promotes bile flow and is a laxative. Take as a decoction, or use a tincture or fluid extract in hot water, allowed to cool. Use as a simple herb or combine with vervain, barberry, and wahoo (*Euonymus atropurpureus*), or fringe tree; or add five drops goldenseal to improve liver function.

When it comes to liver secretions use barberry. For liver toxicity herbs to use are use astragalus, chaparral, or licorice. For engorged liver, use cascara sagrada.

If there is itching of the skin use a lotion with chamomile in it.

Note: there are a number of herbs that may be harmful to the liver. They include: bonset, borage, comfrey, life rot, pennyroyal, sassafras, sweet flag, sweet woodruff, tropical periwinkle and yohimbe.

Woodruff has been used to treat liver and heart problems; it is also supposed to be calming to the stomach. But James Duke reported in the *Handbook of Medicinal Herbs* that test animals suffered "extensive liver damage, growth retardation, and testicular atrophy" when fed coumarin as part of their diet. Coumarin is a constituent of woodruff and it contains woodruff's vanilla scent. (It is widely used in perfumes.)

Be aware that there is some evidence that parsley may be toxic in large doses, causing a decrease in blood pressure and pulse rate, followed by muscle weakness and paralysis. It is also believed that too much parsley may contribute to lung congestion and swelling of the liver.

Part 2: Stomach Problems

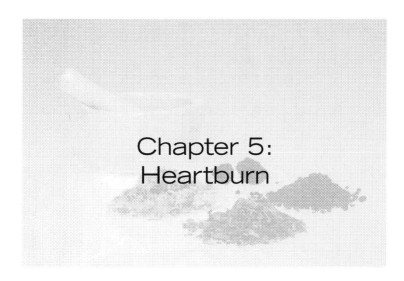

Chapter 5:
Heartburn

I am almost sure everyone has had heartburn at one time or other. What can you do when that burning sensation right under your rib cage won't go away? You belch, but there is no fire department to put out this fire. This is the inferno of that after-dinner heartburn.

The cause of this post-dining firestorm is actually the hard-working sphincter in your lower esophagus. This is a muscle that relaxes to let food pass into your stomach, and then quickly closes. But when it doesn't close properly, the contents of your stomach can back up—a condition known as esophageal reflux—creating a burning or irritation under the rib cage. In pregnant women, and in everyone over the age of forty, the esophageal sphincter is likely to be weakened a bit. There's not much you can do about that.

Regardless of your age or whether you're expecting, the main causes of heartburn are obesity, anxiety, stress, and the wrong diet. Eating the wrong combinations of foods, eating too quickly, eating too much, or missing meals can also attribute to the problem. Those things, unlike your age, are changeable. With proper care, the esophagus can heal from the burning caused by stomach acid within seven weeks, and you can decrease the chances of reoccurrences. Antacids encourage further acid secretion and can actually worsen the condition. If you have heartburn, some key symptoms are bloating and a feeling of abdominal fullness, a burning sensation in your chest, heartburn or acid reflux, and stomach pain.

Conventional Treatments for Heartburn:

The best treatment is prevention. Watch out for foods that tend to bring on heartburn, such as, coffee, alcohol, spicy foods, and citrus fruits. Also be careful when consuming fried and fatty foods, tomatoes, and chocolate. Any of theses foods can irritate the esophageal lining or relax the sphincter muscle, triggering a reflux action.

Do you suffer after a spicy meal with onions? The onions—not the spices—may be the cause. Onions are a common offender. It helps to refrigerate raw onions before you slice them, because it reduces their potency. (They're also easier to digest when cooked.) There are three types of onions that do not cause heartburn: Texas sweet Onions, the Maui, and the Willa Willa varieties. These may not be available in your grocery store, but ask your grocer and he may be able to get them in for you.

Eat small meals to avoid heartburn. It is best to eat somewhat frequently rather than a lot of food all at once. Try to have your last meal of the day at least three hours before bedtime, since you are more likely to get heartburn (esophageal reflux) when you are lying down. Drink water with your meals. Drinking water will wash stomach acids from the surface of the esophagus back into the stomach, and the saliva you swallow with the water will help neutralize the acid. If you think milk helps the problem, think again. It feels good at first because it coats the stomach, but after the milk is digested it stimulates the stomach to produce even more acid, making the problem worse.

Your after-dinner habits may be causing your heartburn. For greater comfort, avoid drinking alcohol, smoking, napping, and strenuous lifting. Smoking weakens the lower esophageal sphincter. Try to resist after-dinner naps, especially after a large meal. Gravity helps food stay in your stomach and intestines where it belongs. Lifting heavy things after eating also brings on heartburn. On the other hand, eating an apple, or having a drink of apple juice after you eat is known to neutralize the acid.

Although exercise is a great habit, running can cause "runner reflux." If this is a problem for you, do other forms of exercise that don't jostle the body as much, right after a meal. Go for a relaxing stroll.

Some medications can lead to heartburn, such as certain high blood-pressure medications. Calcium channel blockers are also known to contribute to heartburn. Medications for inflammation are hard on the stomach, so these should be taken with food if possible. If you are about to pop a couple of aspirin in your mouth, be aware that aspirin, ibuprofen, and products that contain these medicines can burn the esophagus as well as the stomach, warns Dr. Douglas Walta, a gastroenterologist from Portland, Oregon.[3]

You can reach for relief with antacids, but timing is important. It's best to take antacids after you eat *before* heartburn occurs. It appears it is the coating action (rather than the acid-neutralizing action) of antacids that matters. Do not drink water with the antacid, or you may wash the coating away. Antacids come in many forms, including tablets, pills, and liquid. Choose a chewable antacid, because when you chew, you create saliva, which helps neutralize some of the burning acid. Dr. Nalin M. Patel, a gastroenterologist and clinical instructor at the University of Illinois at Urbana-Champaign, suggests taking a dose of antacids in tablet or liquid form about every six hours as needed. But do not exceed the dosage provided by the manufacturer, because excess antacids can cause constipation or diarrhea.

Eating an apple after you eat is also known to neutralize the acid, or have a drink of apple juice.

Herbal Treatments for Heartburn

It has an unappealing name, but vomit nut (*Nut vomixa*) is a homeopathic remedy that relieves heartburn. Your local health-food store might have it, or you can order it online. Just follow the directions on the label.

Florence fennel (*Foeniculum vulgare*) is a carminative and works as an anti-inflammatory; it is effective for griping pain. Take as an infusion or tincture; or take four hundred milligrams of powder in capsules three times a day. Use as a simple herb or add American cranes bill to reduce acidity, or peppermint, meadowsweet, or chamomile to enhance carminative action. If you are pregnant, be wary of high doses of fennel.

Lemon balm (*Melissa officinalis*) is a relaxing carminative; it has a sedative action, which is useful for nervous stomachs. Take as an infusion

---

3   Renner, John, and the Consumer Health Information Research Institute. 1993. *The Home Remedies Handbook by the Editors of Consumer Guide and Hundreds of Leading Doctors.* Louis Weber Publications Int., Lincolnwood, IL, p. 196.

or tincture; add chamomile or meadowsweet as an anti-inflammatory or some hops as a bitter and antispasmodic.

Peppermint (*Mentha piperita*) is a wonderful, soothing herb, and also tastes good. It is a cooling carminative; it stimulates bile flow and is good for nausea and nervous stomachs. It is widely used in hospitals on the surgical units for patients with gas distention and pain. It is also safe for nursing mothers after childbirth, but be aware that it may reduce milk flow. Add fifteen grams of the dried herb to five hundred milliliters of water for an infusion; take up to two and one-half milliliters tincture per dose. Peppermint can be used alone, as a tea, or add American cranesbill to help reduce acid secretions; or marshmallow root, meadowsweet, and licorice to sooth inflammation.

The clinical stomach formula in Appendix 2 is designed to stimulate the digestion and clean out the upper gastrointestinal tract. Meadowsweet stimulates the parietal cells in the stomach to produce hydrochloric acid (HCL)and pepsinogen. By doing this they stimulate the stomach to digest food, and not leave it in the stomach. HCL is used in digestion of food. It is needed for the conversion of pepsinogen to pepsin. Meadowsweet stimulates digestion and cleans out the upper gastrointestinal tract. Pepsinogen is needed to digest protein. Pepsin is a protein splitting enzyme capable of digesting nearly all types of protein. It is formed from pepsinogen in the presence of HCL.

Goldenseal instigates improvements in the quality and quantity of mucus in the gastrointestinal tract, and is called the "king" of the mucus membranes. Fennel and fenugreek seeds aid in the distribution of the mucus. Lobelia helps in establishing autonomic balance; cayenne ensures proper circulation of blood in the stomach area. Some people experience some nausea when taking the mixture. (I blame the cayenne.)

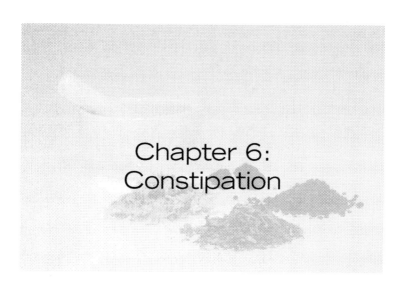

Chapter 6:
Constipation

Do you take *War and Peace* to the bathroom instead of *Reader's Digest*? If so, you are probably constipated. Constipation manifests in two ways. In the first, the sufferer has to strain to move his bowels every time he wants to go. In the second, the sufferer simply just feels the urge too seldom. There is no hard and fast rule about how often one should go, but if you have to go fewer than three times per week and each time it is a strain, there is a good chance you are constipated.

Some resources say that you should have a bowel movement after each big meal you eat. As an example, if you eat once a day then you should go once a day. If you do not eliminate frequently enough, you harbor a lot of parasites and germs that can run rampant in your intestines and these can cause a lot of problems. When the good parasite runs rampid they become bad ones. If you leave a cadaver to root in an enclosed room, this cadaver will be consumed by parasites, which have not been kempt in check by the body. Another bad result is the leaching of toxins into your blood system. It is therefore important to have regular bowel movements and to seek medical advice should a sudden change in bowel patterns occur or if you are pregnant. When pregnant, most women will have a change in their bowel patterns, but if they change significantly for example very constipated, or have diarrhea then you need to see a doctor. Most women become constipated and need medication, or need to eat more fruits and vegetables when pregnant

I have a friend who had part of her stomach removed because she held the food in her stomach too long. Because of this, she was overweight and every calorie she ate was stored in her body. She told me she would only have one bowel movement in a week. This type of pattern is unusual and needs to be managed by a doctor.

Constipation is generally a symptom of other health problems, such as poor diet, sluggish digestion, or lack of muscle tone. It may also result from nervous tension, which in turn inhibits bowel action.

Key symptoms of constipation are a lack of bowel movements for more than twenty-four hours, abdominal pain or gripping pain, which is low in the abdomen, and with difficulty passing stool.

Conventional Treatments for Constipation

A simple way to prevent constipation is to go on a high-fiber diet. Soluble fiber, found in grains, legumes, and fruits, is particularly effective. Oatmeal, rice, wheat germ, corn bran, prunes, raisins, apricots, figs, and apples are also sources of fiber. (Yes, an apple a day *does* keep the doctor away!) Bran cereals are excellent sources of fiber, but when you need a break from them, be sure to eat something to give you the same nourishment. Try other supplements like Fiberall. Be sure to take them with plenty of water, at least six to eight ounces each time.

Always drink plenty of fluids to fuel the fiber. Fluids expand and soften the fiber you are eating, allowing it to form bulk in the colon. That bulking action in turn triggers the urge to move your bowels. Ordinarily, you need to drink about a gallon of fluids a day, but more than that is better.

If you have a problem with constipation, try avoiding milk products, especially cheese, temporarily. Both milk and cheese contain casein, an insoluble protein that tends to plug up the intestinal tract.

Another way to get your bowels moving is to, well ... move! Exercise can help that lazy bowel to function better. Aerobic exercises such as walking, running, and swimming are best for this purpose. If you like to walk, take a brisk walk for twenty to thirty minutes with arms swinging.

Some people who are constipated contribute to their malady by ignoring the urge and waiting until a more convenient time to go. This can aggravate the problem. When your body tells you it is time to go, head for the bathroom. Some people can actually train their bowels to go on a regular schedule at a regular time of the day. Sit on the toilet for about ten minutes after the same meal every day. The key is to stay relaxed. Eventually your body will catch on.

To avoid constipation, avoid what I call water robbers. Coffee, tea, and alcohol are all diuretics that can leave you somewhat dehydrated. Since you need fluids in your system to aid bowel movements, you are more likely to have constipation if you consume these beverages. When you do have them, go for moderation and help compensate by drinking plenty of water. For every cup of coffee you drink, you should drink two cups of water.

Review the medications that you're taking. Medicines that can contribute to constipation include prescription antidepressants and painkillers (especially if they have codeine in them), as well as over-the-counter remedies such as iron supplements, and aluminum-containing antacids. Dr. Marvin Schuster, at John Hopkins University School of Medicine, suggests you keep in mind that the names of most drugs that start with the letter A have aluminum in them. Some medications for high blood pressure are diuretics, which are meant to remove fluid from the body. These also remove fluid from the gut as well. Check with your doctor if you think your medication might be a causal factor in your constipation. Do not quit taking your medication without your doctor's consent.

Not all over-the-counter laxatives are recommended by doctors. In fact, heavy use of laxatives can give you diarrhea, and many are habit forming. If you always rely on a laxative to prompt bowel movements, your body may begin to need it to trigger the action. Laxatives containing castor oil can actually damage your intestinal lining, and those that have mineral oil can interfere with your ability to absorb certain vitamins (especially fat-soluble vitamins like vitamins A, D, E, and K. Some of these vitamins are also needed to absorb nutrients, like calcium. So the laxative can trigger a host of other problems.). "I think laxatives ought to be avoided if at all possible and only used under a doctor's care," says Dr. Schuster. In the long run, you will be much better off by depending on exercise, adequate fluid intake, and a high-fiber diet to keep you regular.

The safest laxatives are the natural or vegetable laxative products. High-bulking agents such as Metamucil, Citrucel, and Prodium, are sold in most drug stores, and if you can tolerate a high-fiber diet, these bulking agents are very safe and helpful supplements. Take a cautionary approach with bulking agents however; follow the directions on the package, increasing the dosage slowly if needed. Not following the directions on the package can cause serious bowel obstructions.

Herbal Treatments for Constipation

For a concentrated constipation buster, go for a fiber supplement that will budge that balky bowel. One of the best is *Psyllium Plantago psyllium/P. Ovata*, which is sold in health-food stores. Add one teaspoonful to a glass of water or juice and stir thoroughly before drinking (you may also make a "paste" of one teaspoon of psyllium moistened with water. Be sure to drink at least one full glass of water afterward). Psyllium is a mucilaginous bulking agent, which lubricates the bowel. It is very useful if the stool is dry. Another way you can take it is by infusing one teaspoon of seeds in a cup of boiling water, let the liquid cool and then drink it along with the seeds, once or twice a day. Use as a simple herb mix with one part linseed to two parts psyllium seed or blond psyllium, if desired. Metamucil, a bowel regulator I mentioned earlier, contains psyllium.

Another good herbal treatment is rhubarb (*Rheum palmatum*). When it is in season in early summer (or if you freeze it, it will be available anytime), fresh rhubarb is a delicious and powerful antidote to constipation. It contains a good amount of fiber, which helps keep things moving. For a rhubarb juice refresher that will get your tract on track, try this cooling recipe: chop three stalks of rhubarb (remove the leaves, which are toxic) and mix with one cup of apple juice, one-quarter of a peeled lemon (The rind is full of vitamin C, which is good for you. It also gives it a stronger lemony taste to it. It also give extra bulk, which is needed for bowel movement) and one teaspoon of honey. Put all the ingredients in a blender or food processor and puree until smooth. This is a good thirst quencher in the summer, as well as a laxative. (Be careful not to drink too much.)

Rhubarb contains anthraquinone, which irritates the digestive tract, increasing gut movement. Another way of taking rhubarb is adding ten to fifteen grams of the herb to six hundred milliliters of water for a decoction; or take two milliliters tincture up to three times a day. Add one to two fennel, and or lemon balm, or chamomile tincture per dose to prevent griping. Enhance with mild laxatives such as butternut or yellow dock. Some caution: take a small amount of rhubarb juice at first and see how your body responds to it. It can be as powerful and quick acting as prune juice. Also, depending on how you like the taste, you might want to mix it with other juices. Note: rhubarb root should be avoided by people with a history of calcium or kidney stones.

Another herb that you might try is guelder rose (*Viburnum opulus*). It is a smooth muscle relaxant and is useful if constipation is linked to visceral tension. Take it as an infusion or tincture. Add laxatives like butternut or licorice, or additional relaxants such as chamomile depending on the symptoms. Use chamomile for cramps, Licorice for smooth muscle relaxant. Black licorice needs to be monitored by a doctor if the person has a heart problem, as the heart is a smooth muscle and licorice affects the heart. Butternut is a laxative it has essential fatty acids that are vital for cell function.

Some animal studies suggest that rhubarb also stimulates uterine contractions, lending some credence to its use in China as a menstruation promoter. Thus pregnant women should try to avoid it. Other women might try it to begin their period.

Other commonly used laxatives are oranges or orange juice from freshly squeezed oranges with the pulp. Beet greens (the leaves of the beet) steamed in a steamer are a good laxative and a good source of iron as well.

For chronic constipation try balm of Gilead. For mild constipation try licorice (the herb, not the confection). Use caution with licorice, as it causes heart palpitations in some people. Although other remedies are available, I've use those listed above and I know they work for most people. However, if you have chronic constipation, have rectal bleeding, or suspect other problems with the bowel do not hesitate to seek medical help. You may be experiencing medical problems other than constipation that can be serious.

Part 3: Reproductive Organ Problems

Chapter 7:
Yeast Infection

It takes very little to get the normally docile *Candida Albicans* fungus (yeast) that lives in a woman's vagina to turn into a rampant troublemaker. Excessive *Candida* is often seen in conjunction with diabetes, getting pregnant, using spermicidal cream or birth control pills, and taking antibiotics. It also occurs in women who have a low immunity to infections, and if you nick the vagina walls inserting a tampon, that can trigger this most common form of vaginitis. Even healthy women usually have this yeast on the skin, and in the mouth, digestive tract, and vagina.

At times the yeast can grow very quickly. While yeast infections can occur at almost any time of life, they are most common during the child-bearing years. Yeast infections are not dangerous as a rule, but they can be painful and embarrassing. When they do become dangerous is when the woman has a very low immunity, and the infection becomes septic (like blood poisoning). You get the same symptoms, for example. aches, chills, and fever. The infection is spread in the blood, throughout the body. Common symptoms of yeast infections include a bothersome itch and burning that can become maddening. Often there is a white discharge that resembles cottage cheese, sometimes accompanied by a yeasty or fishy smell. There may be some vaginal soreness, irritation, or burning, and a rash or redness around the vagina.

If you have consulted a doctor for yeast infections and yet see the symptoms recur, you may be able to save the time and expense of a return visit to the doctor by going to the drugstore and buying a strip of litmus paper or pH paper. Moisten the paper with a small amount of vaginal discharge (the discharge must be wet to react to the paper). If you have a yeast infection, your pH will be between 4 and 4.5 or less, possibly 0.5 or less. If the litmus test confirms your suspicions, you may want to try an over-the-counter drug to treat the malady.

Conventional Treatments for Yeast Infections

As with any disorder, the best thing you can do is avoid it altogether, so I'll first address ways to avoid getting yeast infections.

Eating sugar can cause chronic yeast infections—which is one reason why women who binge on sweets are particularly prone to them. Avoid candy, cakes, pies, and anything with refined, white, or powdered sugar. Diabetics with uncontrolled diabetes or people who excrete high amounts of sugar in the urine also are prime candidates for yeast infections. Yeast loves sugar. If you must indulge your sweet tooth, use brown sugar or honey. Since these take longer to break down in your body, you will lessen the amount of circulating blood sugars, which can trigger yeast infections.

There is also a connection between yeast infections and yeasty foods. To help prevent yeast infections, avoid items likes bread, mushrooms, and alcoholic beverages. People with chronic yeast infections who avoid these foods for three to six months will often notice a significant improvement. Also, eat plenty of foods that are high in vitamin C, such as potatoes, citrus fruits, and broccoli. Vitamin C helps boost your immune system, and if your immunity is down, you are a prime candidate for yeast infections. Diabetics with uncontrolled diabetes or people who excrete high amounts of sugar in the urine also are prime candidates for yeast infection. Yeast loves sugar.

Tight-fitting clothes don't allow for good air circulation in the vaginal area, so stay away from clingy polyester, Lycra, spandex, leather, and other fabrics that don't breathe. Mother knew best when she wore the loose cotton briefs. Yeast thrives in areas that are moist, dark, and warm. If you must wear tight clothing or Lycra, do it for only a few hours—then change into loose-fitting garb made from cotton or other natural fibers. Avoid pantyhose when you can, because they are too restrictive in the vaginal area. Another tip is to quickly change out of wet clothing. When lounging in a wet bathing suit, you are wearing a perfect environment for yeast to grow.

Note that regardless of what type of treatment you use for a yeast infection, if you are a sexually active woman, then you must also consider your partner. This person may be carrying the infection as well and may also need to be treated for it. Until both of you are no longer infected, you will transfer the infection back and forth to each other.

Perhaps the best weapons against yeast infections are in your laundry room, but you have to use special tactics to conquer *Candida Albicans*, because it can survive regular wash-and-dry cycles. The following techniques should help:

Soak panties in water for thirty minutes or more. After soaking them, scrub the crotch of your panties with *unscented* detergent before putting them into the washing machine. Make sure to rinse thoroughly, since residues from soaps and detergents can intensify vaginitis. Another method of ensuring that your underwear is not harboring unwanted yeast is to iron it. Studies have shown that heat-sensitive *Candida* dies when panties are touched up with a hot iron.

Many people find that over-the-counter antiyeast vaginal creams are effective. The creams are available in most pharmacies. Just follow the directions on the package. Avoid bubble baths, scented tampons, colored toilet paper, and other products with dyes, perfumes, and other chemicals that can irritate vaginal tissue. White toilet paper is best.

Another technique is to sit in a sitz bath. Frequent douching should be avoided, since it can be too irritating to those yeast infections. This provides an easy cleansing solution for your vaginal area. Fill the bathtub to hip height with warm water, then add one-half cup of salt (just enough to make the water taste salty), and one-half cup of vinegar. Stay in the sitz for about twenty minutes. Frequent douching should be avoided, since it can be too irritating to the vaginal area, but if you like the douche idea, douche with this solution one tablespoon of salt, and three tablespoons of vinegar put in 2 cups of water. Dr. Sadja Greenwood, a professor in the department of obstetrics, gynecology, and reproductive science at the University of California at San Francisco, has observed that "some women find relief using Lactinex (*Lactobacillus*) tablets vaginally once or twice a day and douching with the vinegar solution twice a day for two days."

Give all applicators (either from the douche or cream) a good scrub. If you use an antiyeast cream you are probably reusing the applicator, so be sure to wash the reusable applicators in hot soapy water. Remember, that to truly heal an infection of the vagina or any other part of the reproductive system, remedies must be used that aid in clearing the infection from the whole body, and cleaning the body as a whole, as most medication taken only clear the symptoms and do not alleviate the underlying problem. Douches or other local applications will at best only get rid of the symptoms for a while.

If you are a sexually active woman, then you must also look at your partner. This person may be carrying the infection as well. So if you treat yourself then you may need to treat that person as well. The infection will be transferred back and forth, from partner to partner.

Herbal Treatments for Yeast Infections

An appropriate treatment for vaginal infections involves the use of antimicrobials in association with herbs that clear the lymphatic vessels usually alteratives. You need to clean the lymph system as well to get rid of infections to aid the healing of infected tissue; astringents will usually be indicated, especially in cases with mucus discharge. The whole picture has to be taken into account and the state of general health as well. If your health is in a state where it cannot take anymore stress, then you can go into a healing crises, which feels like a very bad flu. Then you have to increase the strength of the body before cleaning it. This belief is held by conventional and herbal doctors alike. Yogurt's *lactobacillus* cultures fight the *Candida* bacteria. While some experts recommend inserting the yogurt into the vaginal area, an easier and more accepted way to heal with yogurt is to eat at least ½ cup (containing live cultures) each day to prevent and treat infections. Use plain yogurt for inserting vaginally. Homemade is the best for both applications. Nearly all yogurts contain live cultures. If you don't like the taste of yogurt, you can get a dose of the same helpful bacteria by drinking milk containing live *lactobacillus*. This type of milk will be identified on the container as cultured milk, acidophilus milk, or kefir milk. Plain yogurt, by the way, is also used on some cancer wards for vaginal cancers. It decreases the infections and the odor of the cancer.

One herb that is used for yeast infections is pot marigold (*Calendula officinalis*). It is an antifungal agent and is good for excess yeast in the gut, as seen in candidiasis. Take it as an infusion or tincture, well diluted in water. Add antimicrobials such as purple cornflower, nervines such as lemon balm or an anti-inflammatory like elderflower or agrimony.

Garlic (*Allium sativum*) is another herb that may be used. It too is an antifungal; it supports recovery of the gut flora. Use one clove a day in cooking, or take two two-hundred-milligram capsules a day. This is best used as a simple, or with parsley to reduce the garlic odor. (Note that parsley should be used with caution by women who might be pregnant.) One can easily cover the odor of garlic by sucking on cloves, or by taking chlorophyll or wheat grass juice. Garlic is good for *Candida* because of its antibacterial properties against gram-positive and gram-negative organisms.

Agrimony (*Agrimonia eupatoria*) soothes the gut irritation as well as heals the damaged mucus membranes of the vagina. Take as an infusion or up to four milliliters tincture three times a day. Add lemon and chamomile to reduce stress. Combine with a soothing anti-inflammatory such as marshmallow root.

Other antimicrobials that you might want to use include such herbs as echinacea, or wild indigo. For the lymphatic vessels for this area, herbal treatments include cleavers and poke root. Astringents that may be used include American cranesbill, Beth root, false unicorn root, life root, oak bark and periwinkle. Astringents will prove effective as external applications in combination with tea.

One herb available in a tea form that has anti-inflammatory, antibacterial, antiviral, antineoplastic, and fungicidal properties is lapacho. It has significant antibiotic effects, especially against fungi. Vaginal douches, suppositories, or tampons soaked in lapacho tea have been successful in cases of vaginitis.

A useful mixture to be taken internally is:

2 parts American cranesbill
2 parts Beth root
2 parts echinacea
2 parts periwinkle
1 part cleavers.

This tea should be consumed three times a day. If you use ½ teaspoon to 1 part, make a tea with 2 cups of hot water. Drink 1 cup of tea three times per day.

The mixture may also be used as a douche, made in the same way as an infusion. As a douche it should be used three times a day and should accompany the consumption of the tea, to support the internal treatment. The combination of the tea and douche should be continued for a few days after the infection has cleared.

Chapter 8:
Premenstrual Syndrome

Not too many people need to be told what premenstrual syndrome (PMS) is like. But for those who are lucky enough not to be affected, it's a far cry from sugar, spice, and everything nice! Yeah! What about breast pain, bloating, weight gain, acne, cramping, headaches, food cravings, and mood swings? When it comes to describing the experience of womanhood known as premenstrual syndrome, nice isn't exactly the first word that pops into my mind. PMS's varieties of unpleasant experiences are brought on by fluctuating hormone levels. About half of all American women between the ages of twenty and fifty have PMS. But even though PMS brings on many kinds of discomfort, luckily there are also many treatments.

Finding the best treatment for you, however, may take some experimenting. PMS seems to be affected by stress, doctors say, and they all agree that diet may be a significant contributor. So if the ups and downs of PMS are all too familiar, you might begin by looking at what is on the menu.

The Chinese believe that hormonal imbalances are associated with stagnant qi levels, or energy, around the body. The liver stores blood, and controls the flow of qi. Common PMS symptoms are explained in terms of liver disharmony: irritability because the liver is associated with anger, abdominal bloating is a manifestation of stagnation of qi in the lower abdomen, digestive upsets and sweet cravings occur as a

47

result of excess liver energy invading the spleen and causing deficiency and weakness.

Conventional Treatments for Premenstrual Syndrome

One of the first things you want to do if you suffer from PMS is get the saturated fat off your plate. Eating a lot of fatty foods will increase PMS symptoms and pain. It helps to avoid fatty cuts of beef, lamb, and pork. Better yet, eat poultry and fish as substitutes and replace butter (which is high in saturated fat) with polyunsaturated oils such as flaxseed, corn, and safflower oils.

Limit your salt intake. Food that has a high salt content contributes to fluid retention. Most snack foods and other processed foods are extremely high in sodium, and some boxed cereals and many condiments are higher in salt than many realize. Read the labels on packages; choose fresh fruits and vegetables when possible. Some experts suggest eating foods high in certain key vitamins and minerals to avoid symptoms of PMS. Diuretics, which are taken to decrease the fluid retention during PMS can deplete the potassium stored in the body as well. Potassium is needed for carbohydrate and protein metabolism, and conduction of nerve impulses and contraction of muscle fibers.

Do your skin a favor with vitamins A and D. This dynamic duo plays a part in suppressing PMS acne and oily skin. The best food sources of vitamin A are raw carrots, cooked spinach, cooked sweet potatoes, and fresh cantaloupe. Sunshine provides vitamin D, but you can also get this nutrient from fortified milk and cereals. Feel better with vitamin B6. Increasing your intake of this vitamin can help alleviate symptoms such as mood swings, fluid retention, breast tenderness, bloating, sugar cravings, and fatigue. Supplements of twenty-five to one hundred milligrams per day are well tolerated by most women. Also be sure to eat foods that are high in vitamin B6, which include many kinds of fish and the white meat of chicken and turkey, as well as potatoes and bananas.

Vitamin C reduces stress and allergies; it acts as antihistamine as well. It will be particularly good for those whose allergies tend to act up at this time of the month. Good sources of vitamin C are broccoli, Brussels sprouts, and raw peppers, as well as many fruits and fruit juices.

Some fruits are especially high in vitamin C, including cantaloupe, grapefruit, oranges, and cranberry and citrus fruit drinks.

Another vitamin that has a powerful effect on the hormonal system is vitamin E. This vitamin can help relieve the systems of painful breasts, anxiety, and depression. Food sources for this vitamin are cooking oils and salad dressings, such as olive oil, safflower oil, and corn oil, and a few fruits such as blackberries and apples.

Calcium helps relieve the cramping and pain associated with PMS. Vitamin E is an antioxidant: it prevents the oxidation of vitamin A and polyunsaturated fatty acids. Magnesium also helps with food cravings and stabilizes mood swings associated with PMS. It also plays a role in providing energy for cellular processes. When intake of magnesium is high, a smaller percentage is absorbed from the intestine. Absorption also increases as protein intake is increased, while it decreases as the intake of calcium and vitamin D increases. Sources for magnesium are skim milk (which is great if you are not lactose intolerant), green leafy vegetables, beans, peas, and tofu, and canned salmon, spinach, rice bran, halibut, and mackerel.

Counter the cravings for carbohydrates. Common food cravings focus on sweets and snacks such as ice cream, chocolate, and potato chips. But you will do yourself a favor if you can switch to other kinds of snacks when you get these urges. Eating complex carbohydrates such as whole grains, cereal, and whole-wheat pasta and bagels is probably the best way to ward off food cravings. These foods are a good source of fiber, which helps clear excess estrogen (which has been shown to contribute to PMS) from your body. Cereal and other healthy foods high in carbohydrates actually relieve the psychological symptoms of tension, anxiety, and mood swings.

Have a heaping bowl of unsweetened cereal when you get hungry (remember to chose a low-salt variety). It works like Valium. In general, it is found that women who have PMS are more alert and happier when they eat high-carbohydrate foods rather than high-protein, low-carbohydrate foods.

Go for locomotion to alleviate PMS. When your mood takes a walk on the wild side, you should take a walk as well. Exercise has been found to significantly reduce many physical and psychological PMS symptoms. Dr. Harold Zimmer, an obstetrician and gynecologist in Bellevue,

Washington, concurs with this in *The Home Remedies Handbook*.[4] That is because exercise releases endorphins (brain chemicals) that ease pain and produce a sense of well-being; it also has been shown to reduce breast tenderness, food cravings, fluid retention, and depression. Exercise at least three times per week, even when you do not have PMS. Walking is the exercise of choice; it helps keep bones strong. Go out for twelve to thirty minutes (and longer is better!). I guarantee that you will feel better when you engage in physical activity than when you do not.

Decrease your caffeine consumption to help diminish PMS symptoms (don't tell my mother, because I am a caffeine-aholic). Many foods contain caffeine—coffee, tea, colas, and chocolate, but of course you can instead buy caffeine-free products. Studies have suggested that the risk of PMS is between two and seven times greater in women who consume two or more cups of coffee or tea a day. Caffeine is a stimulant and can contribute to anxiety, irritability, and breast tenderness. Because caffeine is a component of some pain relievers, read labels of pain relievers carefully. If you are unsure about whether your pain reliever has caffeine in it, ask your pharmacist.

Stay on the wagon. Alcohol is both a depressant and a diuretic that can worsen PMS symptoms.

Herbal Treatments for Premenstrual Syndrome

Herbal treatments often center on stimulants and herbs that move the excess liver energy associated with PMS. Modern herbal treatments will often adopt a multidimensional holistic approach—for example; hormone regulators like chaste tree can be combined with uterine tonics such as motherwort or black cohosh to ease menstrual disorders. The kidney is considered (in Chinese medicine) to store the body's vital essence.

In my opinion, the first herb of choice in alleviating the symptoms of premenstrual syndrome would be evening primrose (*Oenothera biennis*). It contains gamma-linolenic acid for prostaglandin production; it eases breast tenderness as well. It helps regulate hormones, both male and female. Take two hundred fifty to five hundred milligrams in capsules

---

4   Renner, John, and the Consumer Health Information Research Institute. 1993. *The Home Remedies Handbook by the Editors of Consumer Guide and Hundreds of Leading Doctors.* LouisWeber Publications Int., Lincolnwood, IL, p. 293.

a day. You can use it as a simple herb, or combine it with other PMS supplements like vitamin B.

Lady's mantle (*Alchemilla vulgaris*) regulates menstrual cycles with a gentle hormonal action; it is also an astringent. Take as tincture or use as an infusion with other herbs. Combine with ten to twenty drops of black cohosh, pasque flower, mugwort, or dong quai tinctures per dose, or add dead nettle or wood betony to the infusion. You should avoid taking lady's mantle if there is a chance of pregnancy.

Bai shao (*Paeonia lactiflora*) balances liver function and soothes liver energy; it also nourishes blood and yin. It is best used in a combination with one other herb or take as a decoction of forty grams to five hundred milliliters of water, in three doses. Mix ten grams bai shao with five grams each of bai zhu, dong quai, chai hu, fu ling, licorice, and one gram ginger. Add five grams Chen pi for breast tenderness. Caution: avoid the above treatment if your symptoms include diarrhea, stomachaches, and chills.

Chaste tree (*Vitex agnus-castus*) acts on the pituitary gland to stimulate and normalize hormonal functions. Take ten drops tincture in water each morning in the second half of the menstrual cycle. It can be used as a simple herb, but can also be combined with others, such as evening primrose oil and vitamin B supplement. Note that high doses should be avoided because they can cause a sensation of ants creeping over the skin. The motherwort formula in Appendix 2 is good for PMS as well.

Other herbs worth mentioning are lemon balm, which is good for depression, nervous exhaustion, indigestion, and nausea. This herb can be used as an infusion or tincture; it is best made with fresh leaves. Cowslip, hops, mugwort, parsley, ragwort, sage, silverweed, stork's bill, woodruff, and wormwood are also effective herbs in connection with the discomforts of PMS. The motherwort formula in Appendix 2 is also for treating PMS.

Chapter 9:
Menstrual Cramps

Almost any woman in the world can tell you what menstrual cramps feel like. People who think, *what is the big deal?* Are clearly either men, or one of the few women who haven't had the experience of menstrual cramps?

When pain is intense, doctors recommend a checkup to make sure that the menstrual cramps aren't caused by something that may require medical treatment, such as endometriosis or a pelvic infection. Menstrual cramps are also known as dysmenorrhea; this may be due to blood stagnation before bleeding starts, or uterine cramps once the flow begins. Basically, menstrual cramps are pain: the pain can appear in the lower abdomen, either before, or at the start of menstruation; it can spread to the thighs or legs; or even to the back. The pain may be accompanied by headache and abdominal bloating; and one's flow may be scanty or have excessive clots. As with amenorrhea there are two general types of dysmenorrhea. Primary dysmenorrhea includes all cases in which no organic disorder is associated with the symptoms, which are presumed to be due to uterine contractions and emotional factors. More than 75 percent of all cases are of this type. Primary dysmenorrhea generally begins before age twenty-five, but it may appear at any time from menarche to menopause. It frequently ends with the birth of the first child.

Since primary dysmenorrhea, occurs in the absence of organic disease, the diagnosis can be made only after a careful medical history is compiled and a special study of the reproductive organs is made to ensure that no disorder has been overlooked. "In some cases, oral contraceptives may be prescribed," states Dr. Harold Zimmer.[5] Because of the effects such drugs have in suppressing ovulation; they prevent the natural production of the hormone progesterone, which is responsible for certain tissue changes associated with the discomfort of dysmenorrhea. However, medication is often less beneficial than emotional support including the easing of any stress at home, school, or work, and reassurance about the worries sometimes associated with menstruation.

Secondary dysmenorrhea comprises all menstrual pain that is due to or associated with an organic disease of the reproductive tract, such as endometriosis, to cite just one example. Secondary dysmenorrhea can occur at any age. Because this type of the illness requires medical treatment, my comments will address only primary dysmenorrheal.

Primary menstrual cramps are hereditary. During the period your uterus cramps up and your sensitivity to that cramping is pretty acute.

Usually primary cramping will lessen if not go away after giving birth.

Conventional Treatment for Menstrual Cramps

Once you have ruled out a disease of the reproductive tract, here are some techniques to maximize comfort and minimize monthly pains. When it comes to drugs, nonsteroidal anti-inflammatory drugs, such as ibuprofen (Advil) work about the best to relieve menstrual cramps, and they may also take the edge off the breast pain and the diarrhea that sometimes go along with cramps. That is because these drugs inhibit the formation of prostaglandins, chemicals that cause muscle cramps and pain. The trick to easing your pain is to take medication at the very onset of pain or discomfort and repeat it every six hours until the pain subsides. Don't save the medication only for severe pain. It will then take more medication to relieve it.

Walk it off. Exercise is a muscle-tension reducer and a mood elevator, and may reduce menstrual cramps by improving circulation in the

5   Renner, John, and the Consumer Health Information Research Institute. 1993. *The Home Remedies Handbook by the Editors of Consumer Guide and Hundreds of Leading Doctors.* Louis Weber Publications Int., Lincolnwood, IL, p. 261.

pelvic organs. If you are walking, strike a pose that is relaxed, one that lets you breathe rhythmically. If your normally brisk pace wears you out during this time, do yourself a favor and slow down.

A warm bath or a heating pad on your belly or the small of your back can relax muscle spasms and ease cramping pain. Be sure that you're experiencing a menstrual problem, because if you're having an attack of appendicitis, heat applied to the abdomen could be fatal. When you are walking outdoors in cold weather, wear a warm jacket that reaches below your hips. That will help keep pelvic muscles warm and relaxed. Stretch your iliopsoas. These are three muscles (major, minor, and iliacus) on both sides of your pelvis, stretching from your lower spine to your femur—the upper thigh bone. Tight iliopsoas have been implicated in a variety of pelvic organ disorders, including painful menstrual cramps. To make it easier to stand up straight and to open the area between your ribs and hipbone, you need to stretch these muscles. One of the best people to help you with this is a professional massage therapist. Here is how to do it when you don't have access to a professional: in a partial side lunge, spread your feet apart and turn your body over the trailing leg, partially bending the knees, and then lunge to the other side and repeat. This stretches the musculature of the pelvic area and the iliopsoas.

Yoga can provide exceptional pain relief for menstrual cramps. Yoga instructors recommend a light routine that stretches and limbers the hips and other joints but doesn't vigorously compress or stretch the abdomen. Strike a diamond pose: sit on the floor with your back erect. Bend your knees, keeping them as close to the floor as possible. Bring your feet together, sole to sole, making a diamond shape with your legs. Keeping your back straight, breathe in, and then slowly bend forward as you exhale. Breathe in and straighten, then bend forward again as you exhale. Repeat several times—feel yourself sink lower with each exhalation.

Another yoga pose to relieve cramps involves curling up into a ball. Kneel, and then sit back so that your buttocks rest on your heels and bend forward to rest your chest on your thighs. Place your forehead on the floor, with your arms stretched in back of you so that your hands are by your feet. If your head doesn't touch the floor comfortably, rest it on your folded arms. Breathe normally, and as you exhale, imagine your body becoming limper and relaxed. If this pose is uncomfortable, you can do a modified version of this pose in a chair. Sit way back in the chair, with your feet flat on the floor, and then lean forward, wrapping your arms around your knees or lower legs. If you find this too strenuous, just rest your arms on top of your knees.

One other technique to ease cramps is to apply pressure to a pressure point located four fingers' width above the inside ankle bone (at the three yin point) on either leg; press firmly for two to five minutes.

Finally, a supplement that's good to alleviate cramps is calcium. It helps maintain normal muscle tone and helps prevent cramps and pain. Aim to consume about eight hundred milligrams a day, the amount contained in about three cups of milk. And be sure you're getting plenty of magnesium. This mineral optimizes your body's calcium absorption and helps decrease menstrual cramps. Good food sources of magnesium are beans, whole grains such as buckwheat and whole wheat flour, salmon, shrimp, tofu, vegetables, and nuts.

Herbal Treatments for Menstrual Cramps

Herbs such as uterine tonics, antispasmodics, and nervines have a lot to offer in the relief of menstrual pains. Try drinking some herbal tea—ginger root tea is particularly effective. To make it, slice a handful of ginger root and simmer it in water for fifteen minutes. And enjoy. Or you can mix equal parts ginger, blessed thistle, and cramp bark. Infuse one teaspoon per cup of boiling water. One to six cups should be consumed. Jamaican ginger is often given with strong cathartics because of its ability to stop the griping pain that can be associated with strong cathartics. Ginger is used to help with circulation. Jamaican ginger has a strengthening effect on both liver and spleen. Ginger is a diffuse stimulant, antispasmodic, and carminative.

Pasque flower (*Anemone pulsatilla*) is also known to help with cramps. It is a nervine, and an anodyne; good for all pains involving reproductive organs. Take up to twenty drops tincture three times a day for symptomatic relief, or add five grams of the herb to five hundred milliliters of water for an infusion. Add ten to fifteen grams of St. John's wort to the infusion. Caution: use only the dried St. John's wort.

Another herb noted for helping in cramps is dang GUI (*Angelica sinensis*). It regulates the menstrual functions, nourishes the blood, and acts as a liver qi stimulant. Dang gui is best used in combinations; add thirty grams of the herb to five hundred milliliters of water for a decoction and take in three doses. Or combine with five to ten grams chai hu, mugwort, bai shao, or with chuan xiong, in a decoction. Dang gui is available in many commercial remedy forms in Chinese herb shops. Avoid in large doses if you suspect you are pregnant. Blue cohosh (*Caulophyllum thalictroide*) is an antispasmodic with a steroidal component that stimulates the uterus; it's good for pain due to blood stagnation. Use a tincture or decoction. Blue cohosh is best used in combinations. Add one to two milliliters skullcap, motherwort, yarrow, false unicorn root, mu dan pi, or chi shao Yao tinctures per dose. Do not use blue cohosh in early pregnancy. It stimulates the uterus and may cause an abortion. It is good for blood stagnation, however.

Black haw (*Viburnum prunifolium*), is an antispasmodic for the uterine muscle; it is a symptomatic remedy for cramping pain. Take twenty milliliters tincture in water, repeat up to three times a day if necessary. Use as a single herb, or with twenty to thirty drops Jamaican dogwood tincture per dose. Black haw is apparently safe in early pregnancy. Other combinations include the clinical female formula mentioned above.

A good approach to managing cramps is the following cramp bark program.

Begin as soon as you know that the menses is about to occur. If it is started a day before, it is even better.

Take two hundred to four hundred milligrams of calcium with one hundred to two hundred milligrams of magnesium taken two or three times daily.

Then take a multimineral: two tablets twice daily. Magnesium phosphate tissue salt (five drops four times daily or four tablets four times daily).

The following formula:
3 parts cramp bark
2 parts blessed thistle.

This formula can be taken either as an infusion (the dosage being one teaspoon per cup and two to ten cups daily), or in capsule form (the dosage here being two capsules, two to ten times daily). The cramp bark formula is one of the best formulas I know of for the menstrual cramps. This next formula is easier to take but not as effective.

Another formula is a mixture of:

2 parts black haw

2 parts cramp bark

1 part pasque flower.

Drink this tea three times daily as needed.

A more common herb in North America is goldenseal. It is specific for uterine contractions and menstrual problems. It also has a wide array of antibiotic effects. In using the fluid extract, make sure you do not get the colorless one; it is not nearly as good as the colored extract.

Chapter 10:
Heavy Menstruation
(Menorrhagia)

Heavy menstruation increases the risk of anemia and if the excessive flow continues over a number of periods, it is advisable to consult a gynecologist to make sure it does not indicate a more severe problem.

The opposite of amenorrhea (no menstrual bleeding), the causes of menorrhagia are as varied as those that cause amenorrhea. They include influenza and other infectious diseases, stress, polyps of the cervical or uterine tissues, hypertension, congestive heart failure, leukemia, blood coagulation disorders, and many others. Menorrhagia may occur during the early stages of a young woman's reproductive life soon after reaching puberty, and medical treatment may be necessary to control the excessive loss of blood. The key symptoms are a flooding of blood, excessive clots, and prolonged bleeding. Menorrhagia also may involve periods that last for more than seven days, and/or a shortened time period between menstrual cycles. It is important to seek medical advice if you experience a sudden or unusual change in menstrual flow.

Conventional Treatments for Heavy Menstruation

To balance the excessive loss of blood, a diet rich in natural iron is essential. In some cases, a D & C (dilation and curettage, a procedure in which the uterine lining is removed) may be necessary. The administration of hormones and other medications, such as iron tablets to correct anemia resulting from the loss of red blood cells, may be necessary as well. If the patient is beyond the age of forty, or if she is finished having children, a doctor might recommend a hysterectomy.

Herbal Treatments for Heavy Menstruation

This excessive flow can be normalized with the use of astringents, which will regulate bleeding without inhibiting the natural process. While most astringents will help those with a special affinity for the uterus and associated tissues are certainly the best to use. I offer quite a few suggestions below, and I advise readers to consider which herb(s) would best apply to their needs.

One treatment can be based on

1 part American cranes bill

1 part beth root

1 part periwinkle.

This tea should be taken three times a day in the week leading up to a period and during the flow itself. If heavy bleeding is an ongoing problem, the tea should be taken once or twice a day throughout the cycle.

Where bleeding occurs in the middle of the cycle (metrorrhagia) or for that matter at any unexpected time the herbs recommended for Menorrhagia will prove useful. However, it is important to establish the cause for intermittent bleeding, in order to identify the most effective uterine tonics.

Chasteberry is often recommended for heavy periods, as is ai ye (*Artemisa vulgaris var. indicus*). The latter is a styptic and warming herb for the meridians and it is especially useful if bleeding is prolonged. Add fifteen grams of the herb to five hundred milliliters of water for an infusion, or take up to two and one-half milliliters tincture three times a day. Add shepherd's purse, self-heal, or han lian cao to a tincture or infusion, or combine with dang gui in a decoction. Caution: do not use ai ye if you suspect you may be pregnant without professional advice.

Pot marigold is said to be a good herb for treating heavy bleeding; it is an astringent with a wide-ranging action for regulating the menstrual cycle. Take as an infusion or tincture. Add one milliliter shepherd's purse (*Capsella bursa-pastoris*), lady's mantle, greater periwinkle, or American cranesbill tincture per dose as additional astringents.

Shepherd's purse is an astringent and an anti-hemorrhagic herb specific for urogenital bleeding; it eases disorders of the root chakra. Take as an infusion or tincture. Add five drops goldenseal tincture per dose or add white dead nettle (*Lamium album*) to an infusion.

White dead nettle is an astringent and antispasmodic; it regulates uterine blood flow and acts on reproductive organs. Take as an infusion or tincture. Use as a simple herb, or combine it with American cranes bill or greater periwinkle.

Another herb worth mentioning is goldenrod. European goldenrod is known to reduce heavy menstrual flow. Steep one ounce of flowering tops of the European goldenrod in a pint of water or teaspoon of sweet goldenrod leaves in a cup of water. (By the way, local application is known to soothe headaches.)

Bayberry is supposed to be one of the most useful herbs around. (In addition to menstrual problems, it is also good for mucous accumulation in the alimentary and respiratory tracts.) Bayberry is used for hemorrhage, especially of the uterus (whether due to miscarriage or other causes). The vagina should be packed with cotton that has been saturated with strong bayberry tea solution. This same therapy is also successful in decreasing excessive menstrual flow. Bayberry also inhibits bacteria. Because of the similarity in their names, bearberry is often confused with bayberry. In this case, it would be okay to mix them up, as bearberry is also good for profuse menstrual flow. It is a diuretic, astringent, and a soothing tonic. Bearberry is useful in diabetes as well as chronic diarrhea; dysentery; piles; and spleen, liver, and pancreatic problems.

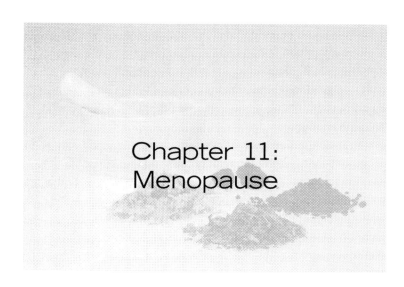

Chapter 11:
Menopause

Another name for menopause is menopausal syndrome. It is associated with hormonal changes and, in Chinese medicine, with kidney qi weakness. Key symptoms are irregular menstruation, mood swings and depression, vaginal dryness, palpitations, forgetfulness, and best of all hot flashes and night sweats. Hypertension and dryness of the eyes are also symptoms that some women experience.

As a woman reaches menopause, (usually around age fifty) hormone levels fall rapidly as the ovaries halt production of the hormone estrogen. Sensing this, the body's internal thermostat tends to react quite strongly. Blood vessels on the skin's surface open up like a radiator, enveloping you in intense heat and flushing your face. About 80 percent of all women experience these hot flashes as they go through menopause. The hormonal changes bring about atrophy of the fallopian tubes, diminished breast size, cessation of menstruation, and even redistribution of body fat.

As I mentioned earlier, in Chinese medicine menopausal symptoms are explained in energy terms and are viewed as a decline in kidney energy. The kidney is considered to store the body's vital essence, or jing. This can be considered the body's life force—a combination of creative and reproductive energies—and menopausal syndrome is explained in terms of kidney energy weakness, affecting both liver and heart functions and causing symptoms such as night sweats, hot flashes, palpitations, back pain, and irritability. In Ayurvedic medicine, the reproductive organs are linked to some of the chakras, or energy centers, within the body. Specifically, the reproductive organs are associated with the root chakras, which in turn are connected to our senses of belonging, or groundedness. Women who are unhappy with their role in life may suffer from reproductive disorders as a physical aspect of this disharmony.

In Chinese medicine, menopausal symptoms are explained in energy terms—as a decline in kidney energy. The kidney is considered to store the body's vital essence or jing. This can be considered the body's life force; a combination of creative and reproductive energies. Menopausal syndromes can be then explained in terms of a weakness of kidney energy, effecting both liver and heart functions. This, in turn, causes night sweats, hot flashes, palpitations, back pain, and irritability. Treatments therefore generally focus on kidney or liver tonics or the use of calming herbs. In Ayurvedic medicine, sexual energy is seen as an aspect of one's creative and spiritual force and should be respected as such. Ayurvedic medicine also sees the reproductive organs as linked to some of the chakras or energy centers within the body, the root chakra being associated with our sense of belonging or groundedness. Women who are unhappy with their lives may suffer from reproductive disorders as a physical manifestation of this disharmony. A hysterectomy can also unsettle the root chakra, leaving some women unable to concentrate, settle, or relax. They seem to have a restless, rootless quality that can be difficult to ease.

Conventional Treatments for Menopausal Syndrome

Your doctor may prescribe estrogen tablets if your hot flashes are severe, but many women find they can deal with milder symptoms with home treatments and a little support from the family.

The first thing you should do is track those flashes. Studies how those hot flashes may occur more predictably and less randomly than you think. To prove it, take note of the date, time, intensity, and duration of the hot flash. Also record the circumstances preceding it—what you ate or drank, and how you felt emotionally.

Some women find that hot flashes worsen when they drink alcohol or coffee, smoke cigarettes, or encounter stressful situations that elicit strong emotions. Your hot flash diary can show you what triggers your need to keep cool.

Lower the temperature. Keeping cool is important for menopausal women since many of the precipitating factors in hot flashes are related to heat. Some doctors suggest sipping cool drinks and wearing natural fabrics that breathe. And one study showed that menopausal women had fewer and milder hot flashes in cool rooms than in hot rooms. So turn on the fan or the air conditioner to keep the temperature down. And when you are going out, carry a fold-up fan with you.

It also helps to keep a cool head—meditate. Some brain research has shown that hot flashes are stimulated by a brain chemical (neurotransmitter) known as norepinephrine, which influences the temperature-regulating center in the brain. This may explain why daily stress reduction practices such as meditation, deep breathing, and yoga, which result in lower levels of norepinephrine, help some women reduce their hot flashes. In one study, menopausal women with frequent hot flashes were trained to slowly breathe in and out six to eight times for two minutes. These women had fewer hot flashes than women trained to use either muscle relaxation or biofeedback.

Your can also douse hot flashes with vitamin E. This nutrient often does a commendable job of relieving the severity and frequency of flashes. Lots of people have good results with it. It is recommended that you start with four hundred international units (IU) twice a day, for a total of eight hundred IU. You should, however, check with your doctor before starting with a vitamin E supplement. While the vitamin is generally considered safe, it can have a blood-thinning effect. Meanwhile, try to include more vitamin E-rich foods in your diet, including wheat germ, wheat-germ oil, safflower oil, whole-grain breads and cereals, peanuts, walnuts, filberts, and almonds.

Get up and go. In one study done in Sweden, severe hot flashes and night sweats were only half as common among physically active postmenopausal women as among benchwarmers. One possible explanation is that exercise elevates the level of endorphins, the feel-good hormones that drop when there is as estrogen deficiency. The endorphins affect the thermoregulatory center—your thermostat. Regular physical activity may increase endorphin activity and therefore diminish the frequency of hot flashes.

Don't be a skinny-Minnie. Estrogen is actually manufactured in body fat from other hormones after menopause. A very thin woman will have less natural estrogen in her system, which may give her more problems with hot flashes. I think I'll stay fat. (I knew there was a reason for it.)

Herbal Treatments for Menopausal Syndrome

Herbal treatments are generally focused on kidney or liver tonics or calming heart herbs. Practitioners of Chinese medicine recommend sipping some sarsaparilla. For centuries, herbalists have used special herbs that have a weak regulating effect on estrogen and may help control hot flashes. The herbs include sarsaparilla, dang quoi, black cohosh, false unicorn root, fennel, and anise. These herbs are available combined in ready-made formulas, or can be used alone. To make a tea, empty one herb capsule into a cup of boiling water and let it steep for a few minutes. Don't drink more than two cups of herbal tea (along with meals is best) daily, and discontinue the herbs if you notice nausea or other symptoms. Talk to your doctor before taking these herbs if you are at risk for cancer or other conditions that rule out estrogen-replacement therapy.

False unicorn root (*Chamaelirium luteum*) stimulates ovarian hormones and can be helpful for early menopausal symptoms after a hysterectomy, or to restart the system after years of contraceptives. Take five to ten drops tincture four to six times a day. It can be used as a simple, or combine it with five drops lady's mantle, two to three milliliters black cohosh, or Mexican wild yam five drops, tincture per dose.

Motherwort (*Leonurus cardiaca*) is a sedative, heart tonic, and uterine stimulant; it is good for palpitations and anxiety. Take as an infusion or tincture. Combine with other sedative nervines like lavender or vervain, or with sage to ease night sweats, or with mugwort. This herb is not advised if you are pregnant.

He shou wu (*Polygonum multiflorum*) is a kidney qi tonic. It nourishes the blood and is useful for menopausal symptoms in older women. It is best used in combinations. Prepare a decoction of fifty grams of the herb to seven hundred fifty milliliters of water, or tonic wine. Combine with nu zhen zhi, gou qi zi, shu di huang, or cinnamon in a decoction. If your symptoms include diarrhea, avoid he shou wu.

Chaste tree acts on the pituitary gland to stimulate and normalize hormonal functions; it can be helpful after a hysterectomy. Take ten drops tincture in water each morning, or take four hundred to five hundred milligrams of the powdered herb. Use as a simple or combine fifteen grams of powder in capsules to relieve hot flashes and other symptoms. Be cautious when using chaste tree, as high doses can cause a sensation of ants creeping over the skin.

Chapter 12:
Hysterectomy

A hysterectomy is the surgical removal of the uterus. In a total hysterectomy, the ovaries are also removed, although most doctors won't do this unless it is absolutely necessary. By leaving a woman with at least one ovary, she will continue to have the benefits of some estrogen production in her body. The word "hysteria" and hysterectomy derive from the same root, and at the turn of the last century, doctors considered the surgery a "cure" for hysteria.

Having a hysterectomy will bring on menopause and indeed, the hormone imbalances characteristic of menopause often go hand-in-hand with emotional and mental turmoil—the "hysteria," if you will. Old herbalist texts will often deal with these problems under the heading of hysteria.

The clinical female formula in Appendix 2 is used to correct hormonal imbalances that can occur at puberty, after pregnancy, at menopause, upon the cessation of birth control, or after a hysterectomy. (In men, the formula can be used in cases of hormonal upsets, especially in the first stages of hormone-related balding.)

Dong quai is a Chinese herb that serves an important role in this formula. This herb is often considered "female ginseng," as it builds up the female organs and regulates hormones the way ginseng does in males. Black cohosh and blessed thistle are Emmenagogues used both to build up and regulate the female reproductive system. Cramp bark's specific function is to reduce cramping in the female organs.

A hysterectomy can unsettle the root chakra, leaving some women unable to concentrate, settle, or relax. They seem to have a restless, rootless, quality that can be difficult to ease.

Women experiencing menopausal syndrome brought on by a hysterectomy are likely to have the same experiences as women whose menopause comes on gradually. In addition to the symptoms mentioned above, they may also experience forgetfulness, irritability, and excitability.

Note that childbirth and certain types of surgery, such as a hysterectomy, can cause pelvic floor muscles to become deficient, and result in incontinence.

Conventional Treatments for Hysterectomy Patients

See the section on menopause for methods of alleviating the symptoms experienced after a hysterectomy.

Herbal Treatments for Hysterectomy Patients

The herbal recommendations that follow would also help with the person who is going through menopause gradually.

My first suggestion is the clinical female formula. This formula has been used very successfully to correct hormonal imbalances that can occur at puberty, upon cessation of birth control pill usage, after pregnancy, at menopause, or after a hysterectomy. You can find the formula in Appendix 2.

Nu zhen zi (*Fructus ligustrum lucidum*) stimulates kidney energy and alleviates symptoms of early menopause. Take as a tincture or use in combination with other herbs in a decoction. Add tonics such as he shou wu, wu wei zi, or ling zhi; add one to two milliliters of rose oil or wood betony tincture for additional support.

Basil is an antidepressant and a tonic for root chakra; it stimulates the adrenal cortex and kidney yang. Eat two to three fresh leaves with salads; take as a tincture or use dilute oil for a massage. Add two drops rose oil to five milliliters basil oil in forty-five milliliters of carrier oil for a massage; add ten to twenty drops pasque flower tincture per dose.

Wood betony (*Stackys officinalis*) is a sedative, it is a stimulant for cerebral circulation and the root chakra, and it eases anxiety and worry. Take as an infusion or tincture. Combine it with lavender, vervain, or basil in tincture and infusion or add ten to twenty drops chaste tree tincture to the morning dose.

Chapter 13:
Prostate Health

Forget about those yearnings for red convertibles and shapely young blondes. The real midlife crisis occurs in a man's prostate, the gland that adds fluid to semen so that he can ejaculate. Four of every five men over age fifty develop an enlarged prostate —or, more specifically, a condition called benign prostatic hyperplasia (BPH). One fourth to one third of them will experience BPH's uncomfortable and potentially dangerous symptoms. BPH usually causes no pain, but it does make urination more difficult. Because the prostate surrounds the urethra, the tube that carries urine from the bladder, it restricts urine flow when it enlarges. This results in a need to urinate more frequently, often with increased difficulty getting started.

With prostate problems, you may also experience dribbling, because the prostate isn't as strong as it used to be and you can't urinate with the same force. Some men with this problem are unable to sleep through the night without waking to urinate, while others are completely unable to urinate—an emergency situation.

A prostate exam is performed quite quickly through the rectum. The doctor can feel the size of the prostate gland and can start treatment accordingly, if necessary. For both enlargement and cancer of the prostate, early detection is vital to a successful cure. That is why it is vital for all men over the age of forty to have regular rectal exams. Your prostate problem may be only an infection, but it may be something more serious.

To reduce an enlarged prostate and improve urination, surgery to remove the prostate is one alternative, and there are several medications to try, although some of them take months to work. But for tried-and-true home treatments here is what you can do.

Conventional Treatments for Prostate Problems:

A good way to ensure prostate health is to cut the caffeine. Caffeine in any form—coffee, tea, chocolate, or soft drinks—tends to tighten the bladder neck and make it more difficult to pass urine. Some of the prostate is made up of smooth muscle, and anything that causes that muscle to constrict will make urination more difficult. Caffeine does this quite a bit.

Alcohol also tightens the bladder neck to hamper urination. And since it is a diuretic, it increases the amount of urine that builds up inside the bladder. Drinking alcohol also makes the bladder operate a lot less efficiently. And the more you drink, the more problems you will likely have. So overindulging in alcohol will not help your urinary tract problems one bit.

Give a cold shoulder to cold medicines. Antihistamines and decongestants can cause even more harm to some men than good. Some men (and women) are more susceptible to the effect of the cold medicine than others. In fact, taking large doses of cold medications occasionally leads to urinary retention, a potentially life-threatening condition in which you completely stop urinating. Decongestants cause the muscle at the bladder's neck to constrict, restricting the flow of urine. Antihistamines simply paralyze the bladder.

If you have allergies as well as prostate problems consult your doctor or pharmacist about prescribing antihistamines. If you must buy over-the-counter medication, take half of the suggested dose. If no problem ensues, move to the full dosage.

With prostate issues, it's best to be wary of spicy foods. Spicy and acidic foods bother some men with enlarged prostates. If you notice more problems after eating salsa, chili, or other spicy or acidic foods, you should avoid them.

Manage your stress. Stress plays a major role in prostate-related discomfort, because the bladder neck and prostate are both very rich with nerves that respond to adrenal hormones. When you are under stress, there are more of those hormones generated and circulating throughout your body—causing more difficulty in urinating.

Stress also triggers the release of adrenaline in your body, prompting a fight-or-flight response. Like it is impossible to get an erection when you are in a heightened fight-or-flight state, it can make urination difficult too.

Get more amours. One way urologists help ease problems is to massage the prostate. For men with mild to moderate voiding difficulties, having more sex can be helpful. Many men notice that the more they ejaculate, the easier it is to urinate. That is because ejaculation helps empty the prostate of secretions that may hamper urination.

Empty your bladder before you go to bed. Many men get the urge to urinate in the middle of the night, and it can be a problem, because it disturbs their sleep and because it can lead to bed wetting. But if you limit your fluid intake after 6:00 PM and make sure you urinate before going to sleep, you can eliminate much of this problem.

Flee south in the winter. If at all possible, spend winters somewhere in the Sun Belt. It is not known why, but people have more trouble urinating and are more likely to go into urinary retention during the cold winter months. Perhaps this is due to an increase in upper-respiratory infections, which many men treat with over-the-counter antihistamines. These drugs tend to aggravate BPH.

A treatment that has been known to work is the combination of glycine, Alanine, and glutamic acid (take two 360-milligram capsules three times daily for two weeks, and one capsule three times daily thereafter). This combination has been shown in many studies to relieve many of the symptoms of BPH. Many companies sell this combination of drugs in a capsule (*prostex.com/feinblatt-bph-article*).

As I mentioned above, prostate problems *can* be more than an inconvenience. An enlarged prostate may cause difficulty urinating, but you shouldn't experience any pain. A somewhat common prostate condition that does lead to pain or discomfort is prostatitis, a bacterial infection that is treated with antibiotics (that is, if you go to a medical doctor, get diagnosed, and treated). If you experience painful urination, coupled with lower back pain, fever, and pelvic pain, you may have a prostate or bladder infection. See your doctor.

Of course it is wise for all men over the age of fifty to see their doctor to be tested for prostate cancer, a leading cancer among middle aged and older men. And if you can't urinate at all, head straight to the emergency room. Urinary retention is extremely uncomfortable and can be life-threatening if left untreated.

Herbal Treatments for Prostate Problems

Buchu is specifically for the prostate and is also a diuretic. For a congested prostate, accompanied by discharge and an aching penis, its therapeutic action is favorable. The herb should not be boiled because of the presence of important volatile oils, when steeped in hot liquid; a covered vessel should be used.

Gravel root is especially valued for its effect on the genitourinary tract. It relaxes and moderately stimulates the tone of the pelvic viscera. As its name implies, it is effective for loosening, dissolving, and eliminating gravely sediment in the urinary areas. It is also used for bloody urine, painful urination, and irritation in the urinary tract. It is also especially valuable for alleviating prostate problems.

Meadowsweet may exhibit some analgesic effect due to its salicylate content. It has also been employed as a diuretic in cases of enlarged prostate, to relieve urogenital irritation. Dosages dried herb: 4.0 to 6.0 gm. daily. As a fluid extract take 0.3 to 1.3 gm. daily, or 0.5 to 1 drams daily, or 1.5 to 6.0 milliliters daily.

White dead nettle is an astringent and a soothing herb with a specific action on the reproductive system, reducing benign prostate enlargement and acting as a uterine tonic. It is useful after prostrate surgery. Take an infusion or up to fifteen milliliters tincture a day. Use as a simple herb or with cornsilk, hydrangea, or couch grass as a healing diuretic and to enhance the action on the prostate.

Saw palmetto (*Serenoa repens*) is a diuretic and a urinary antiseptic with specific hormonal actions on the male reproductive system. This herb reduces benign prostate enlargement. Add ten grams berries to five hundred milliliters of water for a decoction, or take up to two milliliters tincture a day. Use as a simple herb, or combine with hydrangea and horsetail to increase action on the prostate. Saw palmetto is a small, scrubby palm tree native to the West Indies and the East Coast of North America from South Carolina to Florida. Its berries have a long history of use in folklore and have been used for centuries in treating conditions of the prostate. In recent clinical studies, the therapeutic effect of the fat-soluble extract of saw palmetto berries has been shown to greatly improve the signs and symptoms of an enlarged prostate. The therapeutic effect of saw palmetto extract appears to be due to its inhibition of dihydrotestosterone, the compound that causes prostate cells to multiply excessively. Numerous studies on the saw palmetto extract have shown it to be effective in nearly 90 percent of patients, usually in a period of four to six weeks. It is a diuretic so it increases the production of urine. It is also a hormone that can help decrease the size of the prostate. Saw palmetto extract is said to be also less expensive than most other drugs used in the treatment of BPH.

However, very few men will ever hear of the benefits of this herb unless they seek alternative care. They will not hear it from their doctor. The dosage of fat-soluble saw palmetto extract standardized to contain 85 to 95 percent fatty acids and sterol is one hundred sixty milligrams twice a day. If you want the right results, be sure you are using the right extract at the right dosage. Detailed toxicology studies on the extract have been carried out on mice, rats, and dogs, and indicate that it has no toxic effects.

Pygeum (*Pygeum africanum*) is a large evergreen tree native to Africa. The purified fat-soluble extract of the bark has demonstrated clinical efficacy similar to the extract of saw palmetto. However, because the saw palmetto is more effective, that would be my treatment of choice.

The flower pollen extract known as cernilton has been used to treat prostatitis and benign prostatic hyperplasia in Europe for more than twenty-five years. In some double-blind studies, it has been shown to be effective in the treatment of prostatitis due to inflammation or infection. The extract exerts some anti-inflammatory action and produces a contractile effect on the bladder while simultaneously relaxing the urethra. The flower pollen extract is better suited for prostatitis than BPH. The standard dosage for cernilton or similar products is two tablets of five hundred milligrams each, three times a day.

When a man has a bladder infection or inflammation of the prostate gland, the symptoms may not be as localized as that of BPH. Therefore, in addition to the urinary antiseptics the systemic antimicrobial echinacea can be added, and the use of the gonad gland tonic saw palmetto should be considered. This mixture, which appears in Appendix 2, is also used in the case of a swollen prostate gland. Take this mixture three times a day as stated.

Part 4: Pregnancy

Chapter 14:
Early Pregnancy

A lot of changes occur in a woman's body when she is first pregnant. In a nutshell:

First Month:

1. The sperm fertilizes the egg.

2. The egg implants in the lining of the uterus.

3. The mother misses her first menstrual cycle (however, in the first month, some women may experience a small amount of bleeding. If this happens after the first month, you should see a doctor.).

4. The fetus's heart beats regularly (at twenty-four days, but is not audible until sixteen weeks).

5. The fetus's muscles begin to form.

6. Arm and leg buds appear.

Second month:

1. Brain waves from the fetus may be recorded.

2. The lungs begin forming.

3. Ears, earlobes, and eyelids are formed.

4. Permanent fingerprints take shape.

5. The fetus responds to touch.

6. The fetus starts to move.

7. The fetus attains a length of about one and one-quarter inches.

Third month:

1. The fetus moves vigorously.

2. The fetus can hear.

3. The fetus can suck his or her thumb.

4. The fetus begins to hiccup.

5. The fingers can grasp an object.

6. The fetus attains a length of approximately three inches.

Early Pregnancy Challenges

Nausea and vomiting are symptoms in early pregnancy, with some form of nausea occurring in the majority of pregnant women. These symptoms sometimes occur after the first missed period and usually cease by the fourth month. Some women develop an adversion to specific foods; many experience nausea upon arising in the morning; and others experience nausea throughout the day. Many doctors believe that this nausea is caused by hormonal changes in the body, especially the change in human chorionic gonadotropin (HCG). Another theory suggests that changes in carbohydrate needs may create a slight decrease in blood sugar levels in early pregnancy and the nausea may be due to intense hunger. Others think that emotional factors and fatigue may bring on nausea.

Vomiting does not occur in the majority of women.

Another problem in pregnancy is urinary frequency. It occurs in early pregnancy because of the pressure of the uterus on the bladder. This condition usually subsides for a while when the uterus moves out of the pelvic area into the abdominal area, around the twelfth week. As long as other signs of infection do not occur, frequency and urgency of urination are considered normal.

Another problem in the first trimester (which continues throughout pregnancy) is breast tenderness. Increased levels of estrogen and progesterone play a large role in the soreness and tingling sensation felt in the breasts and in the increased sensitivity of the nipples.

Increased vaginal discharge often occurs during pregnancy too. The discharge is usually whitish, consisting of mucus and exfoliated vaginal epithelial cells. It occurs as the result of hyperplasia of vaginal mucosa and increased production of mucus by the endocervical glands. In addition, an accompanying reduction in the acidity of the secretions allows organisms to grow more easily.

Conventional Treatments for the Problems of Early Pregnancy

Treatment of nausea and vomiting are not always successful, but the symptoms can be reduced. It is important to assess when the nausea and vomiting occurs to be helpful in suggesting methods of relief. For some women, nausea may be relieved simply by avoiding the odor of certain foods or other conditions that precipitate the problem. If nausea occurs most frequently during the morning, the woman can be encouraged to try various simple remedies, such as eating dry crackers, dry toast, a piece of matzo, or a plain, unbuttered bagel, before arising in the morning. In general, it is usually helpful to eat small but frequent meals, and to avoid greasy and highly seasoned food.

Some women find unusual remedies that they claim to be helpful and as long as these remedies are not harmful to their pregnancies, that's just fine. For example, you may find that it is easier on your tummy to drink fluids rather than to eat solid food and if that's the case, you can get all your nutrients from liquids.

A number of physicians recommend vitamin B6 for morning sickness because of its ability to fight nausea. Talk to your doctor, however, before trying any supplements. Be sure not to exceed twenty-five milligrams of the vitamin each day.

If you succumb to vomiting, take good care of your teeth and brush afterward. Otherwise, the frequent contact with the harsh acids in what you throw up can eat away at tooth enamel.

Go nuts over almonds. They are high in vitamin B and contain fat and protein—what you and your baby need right now. And they help fulfill the requirement of eating small meals.

Stress makes morning sickness worse, which is one reason why so many working moms suffer from morning sickness. Regardless of whether you have to report to a boss at the office or a grump-prone spouse at home, lots of walking is recommended as a stress reliever. It is also highly recommended for alleviating morning sickness, even if you were sedentary before getting pregnant.

Relieve pressure with acupressure. A daily all-over body massage might be ideal, but in the meantime a little acupressure can do a lot to reduce or cure morning sickness. Ask for your partner's help, as follows: either sit or lie down on your side, with your partner behind you. Have him press his thumb down your back, first following the groove between your shoulder blade and your spine, then keeping up the thumb pressure around the perimeter of your shoulder blade, moving out toward your side. Keep the pressure on for five to seven seconds at intervals along this path. The pressure should be comfortable. If you feel a sore spot, ask your partner to keep his thumb there, giving that spot extra attention. Do the massage three times. Repeat the procedure down the right side. If you stimulate the external, you may eliminate the internal discomfort.

Lift an hourly glass. Getting extra liquids is important, especially if you have been vomiting, so drink several ounces of clear broth, water, fruit juice, or flat ginger ale or cola every hour or so. At the drug store look for Emetrol, a high-carbohydrate nonprescription drink. Emetrol helps calm the emetic center, the portion of your brain that controls nausea. Sports drinks, like Gatorade, are also good, because they replace the electrolytes that are lost when you vomit.

Generally, nausea and vomiting cease by the fourth month of pregnancy. If they do not, extreme morning sickness (hyperemesis gravidarum) may develop, which may even require hospitalization. For some women who suffer extreme nausea and vomiting in the first trimester, an antiemetic may be ordered by the doctor. Antiemetic should be avoided if at all possible during this time because of possible teratogenic effects on the development of the embryo.

There are no methods of decreasing the frequency and urgency of urination in pregnancy. However, fluid intake should never be decreased in attempts to prevent frequency. The leaking of urine during pregnancy is usually limited, unless there is excessive relaxation of the muscles. The muscle tone is believed to gradually weaken with each pregnancy, and bladder problems can occur in older women if perineal muscle tone is not maintained. Tightening of the pubococcygeus muscle, which can be achieved by Kegel exercises, can help maintain good perineal muscle tone. The function of the pubococcygeus muscle is to support internal organs and control voiding.

One simple way to manage breast tenderness is a supportive, well-fitted bra. It gives the most relief for this discomfort.

Cleanliness is important in preventing excoriation and vaginal infections that may in turn be associated with increased vaginal discharge. Daily bathing should be adequate, and douching should not be done at all in pregnancy. If vaginal infections occur consult your obstetrician. Nylon underpants and pantyhose should be avoided, because they retain heat and moisture in the genital area—absorbent cotton underpants should be worn to help prevent problems. Bath powder is also helpful in maintaining dryness and promoting comfort. The pregnant woman should be encouraged to report to her doctor any change in vaginal discharge and any irritation in the perineal area.

Herbal Treatments for the Problems of Early Pregnancy

For generations, herbal remedies were the only option for easing the ills of pregnancy and trials of childbirth but there are some herbs that you shouldn't take if you are pregnant. Herbs to avoid are: aloe vera, juniper, mandrake, parsley, parsley root, pennyroyal, sassafras, and herbs in the *Artemisia* genus, including: mugwort, sagebrush, and wormwood. Although nowadays we are far more cautious about using herbs during pregnancy, they still have an important role to play. As a rule, they provide a safe alternative to allopathic drugs (which can be harmful).

Butternut, for example, is a suitably gentle laxative; nettle tea, watercress, or burdock can help anemia, while powdered slippery elm or marshmallow root will ease heartburn (which most often appears in the third trimester).

Morning sickness is often best treated with a variety of remedies; women who feel sick much of the time may find that a repeated treatment may increase nausea over time.

Some herbs that are safe for pregnant women are raspberry and blackberry. These quiet the nerves and relieve abdominal cramps due to intestinal disturbance (as well as menstrual cramps—they relax the uterus and quiet excessive ovarian action). They are used often to prevent abortion due to nervous afflictions.

Black horehound (*Ballota nigra*) is a good herb for morning sickness. It prevents vomiting, serves as a sedative, and is useful for nervous dyspepsia. Take up to two milliliters tincture in hot water up to three times a day, or sip a weak infusion. Alternate its use with other remedies if symptoms persist.

Roman chamomile (*Chamaemelum nobile*) reduces feelings of nausea and calms the stomach; it is a suitable relaxing Nervine in stressful situations. Drink one cup infusion before rising or take five to ten doses of a tincture as required (up to five milliliters a day). Best as a simple herb, but you can alternate its use with lemon balm, fennel, basil, ginger, or peppermint if need be. It is important to not exceed the dosage stated above.

Ginger (*Zingiber officinale*) prevents vomiting and has been used successfully in hospital trials involving hyperemisis gravidarum patients. Take up to one gram powdered herb in capsules per dose, or take two to five drops tincture as required (up to one milliliter per day). Ginger is most effective when used alone, but it can be alternated with other remedies as required. Ginger is recommended for early pregnancy, and it is important not to exceed the stated dose.

In Chinese medicine, many uterine bleeding disorders can be attributed to a weakness in the Chong (vital) and ren (responsibility) channels—what we regard in the West as acupressure meridians. The ren channel is regarded as being closely related to the yin channels in the body and is also called the "conception vessel," as it starts in the uterus. The Chong channel (which also starts in the uterus) communicates with all the other channels. These channels are associated with childbirth, and any "coldness" and deficiency here can lead to bleeding during the pregnancy. Treatment for women who experience mild bleeding consists of herbal capsules containing dang gui, shu di huang, ai ye, bai shao Yao, licorice, and chuan xiong to warm and nourish the different deficient channels.

Some herbal cosmetics and remedies, such as those made with ginseng, can have steroidal effects similar to those of estrogen. If you suspect that a product that you use may have such an effect, try discontinuing its use for a while to see if the problem, like breast tenderness, improves.

Chapter 15:
Late Pregnancy

It is very difficult to classify discomforts as specifically occurring in the second or third trimester, since many problems are associated with variations in individual women. The conditions discussed in this chapter usually do not appear until the third trimester in primigravada (women who are pregnant for the first time) but do tend to occur earlier with each succeeding pregnancy.

Heartburn is the regurgitation of acidic gastric contents into the esophagus. It creates a burning or irritating sensation in the esophagus and radiates upward, sometimes leaving a bad taste in the mouth. It can occur at any time in pregnancy, but is most common in the second half. Heartburn appears to be primarily a result of the displacement of the stomach by the enlarging uterus. Pregnancy is accompanied by a decrease in gastrointestinal motility and a relaxing of the cardiac sphincter, which also contributes to heartburn.

Most women experience ankle edema in the last part of their pregnancy because of the increasing difficulty of venous return from the lower extremities. Prolonged standing or sitting, and warm weather increase the edema. Ankle edema becomes a concern only when accompanied by hypertension or proteinuria (greater than normal amounts of protein in the urine), or when the edema is not postural in origin.

Ankle edema is also associated with varicose veins. Varicose veins are a result of a weakening of the walls of the veins or faulty functioning of the valves. Some people have an inherited weakness in these walls. Poor circulation in the lower extremities predisposes women to varicose veins in the legs and thighs. With poor circulation, the valves of the legs prevent the blood from going downward, and stasis of the blood exerts pressure, with gradual weakening of the walls, resulting in varicosities in the veins. In other instances, faulty functioning of the valves results in pooling of blood in the lower extremities with concomitant pressure on the vein walls. Occupations requiring prolonged standing or sitting contribute to congestion of blood in the lower extremities. The weight of the uterus and baby in the pelvis aggravates the development of varicose veins. It does this by preventing good venous return. Most women who do not have any of the other predisposing factors can avoid the development of varicose veins through good preventative measures. The signs and symptoms of varicose veins are aching and tiredness in the lower extremities, with the discomfort increasing throughout the day. Sufferers frequently get discouraged by the discoloration in the veins of their legs and obvious blemishes.

Hemorrhoids are varicose veins around the lower end of the rectum and anus. In the nonpregnant state, hemorrhoids are caused by the straining that occurs with constipation. When a woman gets pregnant, the baby and uterus create pressure on the veins and thus interfere with venous return. As the pregnancy progresses and the fetus grows, greater pressure on the veins and greater displacement of the intestines occurs, increasing the problem of constipation and often resulting in hemorrhoids. You might not notice them until the second stage of labor, when the hemorrhoids appear as you strain for a bowel movement. These hemorrhoids usually disappear after the child is born. However, women who have hemorrhoids when they're not pregnant usually experience more problems with them during their pregnancy.

Symptoms of hemorrhoids include itching, swelling, and pain, as well as hemorrhoid bleeding. Internal hemorrhoids are located above the anal sphincter and are usually those that are responsible for the bleeding.

Constipation is another problem when you are in the second and third trimester. The pregnant mother has general bowel sluggishness caused by increased steroid metabolism and displacement of the intestines, which increases with the growth of the fetus. In addition, she may be taking oral iron supplements, which can exacerbate constipation.

Backache is another problem acquired with pregnancy. As the uterus enlarges, increased curvature of the lumbosacral vertebras occurs. The steroid hormones cause a softening and relaxation of pelvic joints; thus the growing uterus stretches the abdominal muscles, and the increasing weight creates a gradual tilt of the anterior portion of the pelvis. As the anterior portion of the pelvis tilts downward, the spinal curvature increases. If the woman does not learn how to correct this curvature, the strain on the muscles and ligaments will cause backache.

Leg cramps are painful muscle spasms in the gastrocnemius muscles (the big muscles located in the back of your calves). They occur most frequently at night when the woman has gone to bed, but may occur at other times. Extension of the foot can often cause leg cramps, so the pregnant woman should be warned not to do this too hard while doing exercises for childbirth preparation or when she is resting. It has been suggested that the leg cramps are due to an imbalance of the calcium to phosphorus ratio in the body, but this idea is still very controversial. Leg cramps are more common in the third trimester because of the increased weight of the uterus on the nerves supplying the lower extremities. Fatigue and poor circulation in the lower extremities contribute to this condition.

Faintness is experienced by many pregnant women, especially in warm, crowded areas. The cause of faintness is a combination of changes in the blood volume and postural hypotension due to venous pooling of blood in the dependent veins. A sudden change of position or standing for prolonged periods can cause this sensation, and fainting can occur.

Shortness of breath occurs as the uterus rises into the abdomen and causes pressure on the diaphragm. This problem worsens in the last trimester as the enlarged uterus presses directly on the diaphragm, decreasing vital capacity. When lightening occurs in the last few weeks of pregnancy in the primigravada, the expectant mother will experience considerable relief. Because women who have been pregnant previously do not usually experience lightening until labor, shortness of breath will continue throughout their pregnancy.

Conventional Treatment of Late Pregnancy Problems

Behaviors that aggravate heartburn are overeating, ingesting fatty and fried foods, and lying down too soon after eating. These situations should therefore be avoided. The woman should be encouraged to eat smaller and more frequent meals to accommodate the decreased size of her stomach area. Antacids such as Amphojel and Maalox can be used to alleviate heartburn. Surprisingly, common household remedies such as baking soda should *not* be used, as it may result in a potential electrolyte imbalance.

Ankle edema can be avoided (and should be as much as possible). If the woman has to sit or stand for long periods of time, frequent dorsiflexions of her feet (moving the toes up toward the shin) will help contract muscles, thereby squeezing the fluid back into circulation. Tight garters or other restrictive bands around the leg should not be worn. During rest periods, the woman should elevate her legs and hips as described in the following discussion of varicose veins.

For varicose veins, preventive and relief measures include frequent elevation of the legs. One important habit that the pregnant mother can develop is to always elevate her legs when she sits down. If you are pregnant, sit with your feet above your hips when possible. A more effective method you can use to promote venous return is to lie on your back on the floor or bed with your legs resting at right angles against the wall (in other words, lying on the floor with your feet on the seat of the chair).

A pregnant woman should not sit for long periods of time or cross her legs at the knees, because of the pressure on her veins. She should avoid standing for long periods of time. However, supportive stockings may be extremely helpful, depending on the amount of discomfort. Supportive stockings should be put on upon rising in the morning and should be washed by hand to retain their elasticity.

Treatment of varicose veins by injection or surgery is not recommended during pregnancy. However, surgery may be necessary after the delivery of her baby, because the problem will be aggravated by each succeeding pregnancy.

Phlebothrombosis and thrombophlebitis are possible complications of varicose veins, but they usually do not occur in healthy pregnant women. If these complications occur, the cause is usually a local injury.

Vulvae varicosities may also be a problem in pregnancy, although they are less common than varicose veins in the legs. Varicosities in the vulva and perineum cause aching and a sense of heaviness in these areas. Support in this area promotes relief. Elevation of only the legs aggravates vulvae varicosities by creating stasis of blood in the pelvic area. Therefore, it is important that the pelvic area also be elevated to promote venous return into the trunk of the body. More than one firm pillow under the hips may be needed to accomplish this elevation. Near the end of the pregnancy, this position may be extremely awkward; the woman may relieve uterine pressure on the pelvic veins by resting on her side.

Hemorrhoids are varicose veins around the lower end of the rectum and anus. Relief can be found by gently reinserting the hemorrhoid with the use of a lubricating ointment. Reinsertion is aided by gravity; therefore, reinsertion is more successful if the woman lies down on her side or in the knee-chest position. External hemorrhoids are located outside the anal sphincter. They are not usually the source of bleeding or pain; however, thrombosis of these hemorrhoids can occur, and in that case they become extremely painful. The thrombosis may resolve itself in twenty-four hours, or it can be treated in the doctor's office by incising and evacuating the blood clot. Avoiding constipation is an important factor in preventing and/or relieving the discomfort of hemorrhoids. Relief measures for existing hemorrhoid symptoms include ice packs, use of topical ointments and anesthetic agents, and warm soaks.

Constipation intervention is discussed in the chapter on constipation. Any woman who develops good eating habits during pregnancy will be prepared to maintain good bowel functions after delivery as well. The woman should not become dependent on laxatives during pregnancy, but they should be taken if needed. Note, however, that using laxatives can become a habit that will need to be carried on after delivery if good eating habits are not maintained.

Backache can be avoided with exercise, and if proper body alignment is maintained throughout pregnancy, backache can be relieved or even prevented. An exercise called the pelvic tilt can help restore proper body alignment. As the anterior pelvis is tilted upward, the curvature of the back is automatically decreased, relieving much of the discomfort.

You can perform the pelvic tilt as follows: while lying on your back, put your feet flat on the floor with your knees in the air to help prevent further strain and discomfort. You relieve the curvature in your back by pushing the raised area toward the hard surface. You (or your partner) can place your (or your partner's) hands under your back to feel the change in body alignment. It is then easier to apply the pelvic tilt when you are standing with your back to the wall and to maintain this body alignment throughout the day. The pelvic tilt includes the simultaneous movements of tightening the buttocks and abdominal muscles, and then tucking under the buttocks. The exercise can be performed on hands and knees and done while sitting in a chair.

The application of proper body mechanics throughout pregnancy, in conjunction with proper posture, is also important. If you're pregnant, don't curve your back by bending over to lift or pick up items from the floor. The strain is felt in the muscles of the back. (This goes for anybody pregnant or not, male and female alike.) Always use leg muscles to do the work. Keep your back straight by bending your knees to lower your body into the squatting position. Your feet should be placed twelve to eighteen inches apart to maintain your balance. When lifting heavy objects such as your child, you should place one foot slightly in front of the other, keeping it flat on the floor and lowering yourself to the other knee. The object is then held as close as possible to your body for lifting. This same principle of keeping the back straight and bending the knees applies when you sit down or get up out of a chair. If proper body alignment is maintained throughout pregnancy, backache can be relieved or even prevented.

Work heights that require constant bending of the back can contribute to backache and therefore should be adjusted as necessary. This applies to the height of what you are working on, whether it is a computer or table, or just a counter. If you need to constantly bend (whether you are pregnant or not) it contributes to back pain. Women who do not experience backache in pregnancy may become aware of it as they bend to change a newborn's diaper in the days and weeks after they give birth.

Immediate relief of muscle spasms in the legs or leg cramps is achieved by stretching the muscle. This is most effectively done by lying on your back and having another person press your knee down to straighten your leg. Foot flexion techniques, massage, and warm packs can be used to alleviate discomfort from leg cramps.

Milk may help alleviate legs cramps; however, drinking large quantities of milk increases the calcium/phosphorus imbalance in the body because of the large quantities of phosphorus that milk provides. The high phosphorus levels depress the serum calcium levels. Therefore, doctors might recommend that the woman drink no more than a pint of milk a day and take calcium lactate as a supplement, or a doctor might allow a quart of milk a day and prescribe aluminum hydroxide gel. Aluminum hydroxide gel stops the action of phosphorus on calcium by absorbing the phosphorus and eliminating it directly through the intestinal tract. The treatment recommendations depend on the frequency of the leg cramps.

When planning a treatment regimen, one must be careful not to totally exclude milk from the woman's diet because it is excellent source of other essential nutrients.

Faintness is experienced by many pregnant women. If faintness is experienced from prolonged standing or from being in a warm, crowded room, you should lower your body to a sitting position, with your head lowered between your legs. If this procedure does not help, you should be assisted to an area where you can lie down and get fresh air. When arising from a resting position, you should move slowly.

Shortness of breath occurs as the uterus rises into the abdomen. During the day, relief can be found by sitting straight in a chair and by using proper posture when standing. If distress is great at night, you can sleep propped up in bed, with several pillows behind your head and shoulders

Herbal Treatments for Late Pregnancy Problems

Squaw vine's most common use is as a parturient, which is how Native Americans used to use it. Mixed in equal parts with red raspberry leaves and in infusion form, it is taken two to four weeks before the expected delivery date to ensure a safe and easy delivery. The dosage is one teacup full, two to three times a day. It is also used in several female corrective tonics. A formula for sore nipples associated with breastfeeding is as follows:

2 oz. squaw vine (as fresh as possible)

8 oz. olive oil.

Beeswax as it depends on what form the beeswax is in as to how long to reduce it. But it should be the consistency of that of a soft salve.

Mix the herb in one pint of water, strain, add oil and beeswax, and slowly reduce until the consistency is that of a soft salve. Apply.

Raspberry leaves are very beneficial during pregnancy. Every expectant mother should drink at least one cup of raspberry leaf daily. This helps make for an easier pregnancy, delivery, and recovery. Most importantly, it helps prevent tearing of the vaginal orifice during the birth, and tones the uterus. Take raspberry leaves as an infusion. One cup a day, in the last two months of pregnancy. Drink plenty of this herb during labor. You can use this herb as a simple herb, or add rose petals and wood betony to infusion during labor.

The clinical female formula noted in Appendix 2 is good for the commencement of labor. If the nervous system is tired, it will relieve the rigidity of the uterus, and calm nervous irritability

Herbs have been used to help the body prepare for childbirth by toning the uterine muscles. The uterus can be prepared for the exertions of birth with tonic herbs or diluted sage oil massaged into the abdomen during the last three weeks. After the birth, basil and motherwort tea can help clear the placenta.

Tears in the peritoneum can be painful and slow to heal. These herbs will also help bruising and soreness. Some tears require stitches if an episiotomy is not performed. In that case these herbs will work on the sutured area. Arnica salve or a tincture applied externally to swollen and painful areas will relieve much of the bruising and pain. Apply the tincture every two to three hours. A salve can be made by heating one ounce of the flower with one ounce of cold-pressed olive oil in a water bath for a few hours. Strained, it is good also for chapped lips, inflamed nostrils, bruises, joint pain, skin rash, and acne.

St. John's wort (*Hypericum perforatum*) is an anti-inflammatory, a healing herb, and an astringent. Apply the infused oil or add a strong infusion to a hip bath. Add lavender and marigold oils to infused oil, or add the dried herbs to infusions for baths.

Pilewort (*Ranunculus ficaria*) is an astringent herb. You apply it as a cream to the effected area. This herb combines well with witch hazel. Caution: this mixture is not to be taken internally.

Comfrey (*Symphytum officinale*) is a healing herb. It encourages cell growth and can help limit scar tissue. Apply as a cream or infused oil or ointment to affected areas, or add an infusion to a hip bath. Mix two milliliters lavender oil in twenty milliliters infused oil base. Because comfrey can cause rapid healing, be sure you only apply it to a clean wound.

Part 5:
Life and Lifestyle

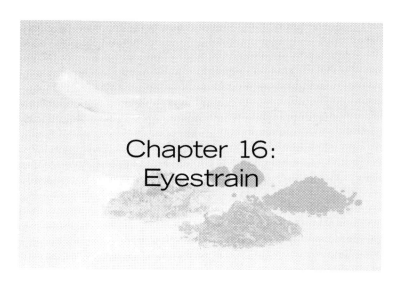

Chapter 16: Eyestrain

Eyestrain can happen to anyone and in fact, almost everyone experiences it, especially by the time he or she gets to age forty. You are likely to have eyestrain at least occasionally from driving, smog, watching television, or staring at your computer. You know you have eyestrain when clear images begin to look blurry. Your eyes start to ache so much that you just want to close them for a while. Here are some ways you can put a lid on eyestrain (other than getting new glasses, which may not be a bad idea if the discomfort continues for a period of time).

Conventional Treatment of Eyestrain

Try time-outs from close work (sounds like a discipline problem, doesn't it?). When you are using a computer or doing any other type of close work that strains the eye, stop every hour for about two minutes and give the eyes a rest. Just close them and do nothing for two minutes. When you are reading, stop every few minutes. There is a muscle in your eye that contracts when you are doing close work; by refocusing, you relieve the spasms in that eye muscle. If you want something to look at, hang a sheet of newspaper on a far wall and try to read the larger print.

If you use a computer, you have probably discovered how important it is to reduce the glare on your computer screen in order to minimize eyestrain. The intensity of the surrounding light is not as important as the positioning of the light source. The light source should be close enough so that is comfortable, but far enough that it does not shine on your screen or into your eyes. Of course, special glare shields on the computer screen help as well.

A few less-well-known secrets include the following tips.

Adjust your computer monitor so that the letters on the screen are at least five times brighter than the background. When buying a monitor, choose one that allows you to choose the color of the type. Type that is amber or green is easiest on the eyes. Screen size is not particularly significant, but letter size is—capital letters should be at least one-eighth-inch high.

Avoid overhead florescent lighting when using your computer, because its flickering can interact with the flicker on your computer screen, causing eyestrain. Even though you cannot see the fluctuation in light, a florescent tube actually flickers about sixty times per second. The computer screen also flickers. When both are flickering it can cause a lot of eyestrain.

Put your eyes on the blink. Your eyes have their own personal masseuse—the eyelids. Make it a point to consciously blink your eyes and not squint. Each blink cleanses your eyes and gives them a tiny little massage. The eyes blink less frequently when using the computer, says Dr. Arnold Prywes, a clinical assistant professor of ophthalmology at the Albert Einstein Medical College in New York.[6] When you are doing close work or concentrating on a computer screen for long hours, remember to blink frequently.

Of course, you should get glasses if your need them. A lot of eyestrain is the result of vanity—obviously, you are going to strain your eyes if your vision is in need of correction, so get a pair of glasses. Or put them on if you have them.

Exercise your eyes. Standing about five feet from a blank wall, have someone toss a tennis ball at the wall and try to catch it as it bounces off. Or hold your thumb out at arm's length. Move it in circles and back and forth as you bring it closer to your face, then farther away, as you follow it with your eyes. Both exercises help offset damage caused by eyestrain and improve the brain-to-nerve muscle connection of you vision.

---

6   Renner, John, and the Consumer Health Information Research Institute. 1993. *The Home Remedies Handbook by the Editors of Consumer Guide and Hundreds of Leading Doctors.* Louis Weber Publications Int., Lincolnwood, IL, p. 145.

Herbal Treatments for Eyestrain

Take a tea break. Warm eyebright tea is a gentle balm for the eyes that are strained. Take a towel and soak it in a brewed eyebright tea. Lie down, place the warm towel over your closed eyes, and leave it on for ten to fifteen minutes. It will make your eyestrain go away quickly. Be very careful not to let the towel drip tea into your eyes, and be sure the tea has cooled down sufficiently before you soak the towel in it. As the name suggests, eyebright is an herb with a long history of use in the treatment of almost all eye diseases. Its botanical name, *Euphrasia*, comes from the Greek word meaning "good cheer," recalling the gladness felt by those who had their eyesight preserved by this plant. The plant owes its use for pinkeye, or conjunctivitis, to its astringent and anti-inflammatory properties. If you see this plant, it often resembles a bloodshot eye, an indication that this plant is good for sore eyes.

Tired, strained eyes can also be soothed by eyecups of rose water or a weak infusion of pot marigold, cornflower, or strawberry leaves. Put one tablespoon of the dried herb in half a liter of water, boil it for ten minutes, and let cool. You can either use it as eyewash or apply it as a compress by misting cotton wool gauze or muslin in the warm liquid and placing it over the eyes for about fifteen minutes. This should be repeated several times a day. If you have an infection, be aware that it needs to be treated internally as well as externally.

Goldenseal (*Hydrastis canandensis*) has made its way into modern medicines. Many manufacturers have included the alkaloid that is extracted from the root in eye drops for inflamed eyes. Several sources, including *Magic and Medicine of Plants,* by the Reader's Digest editors, and *Textbook of Modern Herbology,* by Dr. Terry Willard, recommend celedine as being good for blurred vision and sore eyes. It can be made into oil or an ointment and used in the eyes. If all else fails and you have no herbs around, make some regular tea (Earl Grey or any other type is fine). Drink the tea and relax. Then take the cooled, not cold, tea bags and put them on both eyes. This treatment is also good for welder's flash (caused when a surge of UV light hits the eye).

If you believe that you may have a foreign body in the eye or an infection, it is a good idea to see an ophthalmologist.

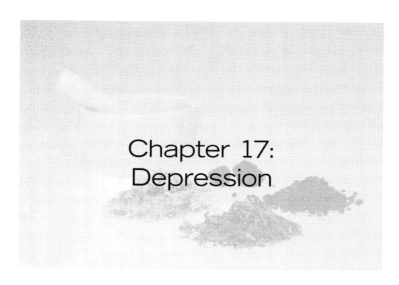

Chapter 17: Depression

Depression used to be such a verboten subject that people often felt compelled to fake a smile and keep their feelings inside. Some people still do. However, since researchers started to discover the mix of psychological and physical causes for this problem, depression has seemed much less mysterious and forbidding. People are acknowledging it and talking about it out in the open.

There is even something called healthy depression, according to Dr. Ellen McGrath, former chairperson of the American Psychological Association's National Task Force on Women and Depression. Dr. McGrath is the author of *When Feeling Bad Is Good,* which discusses in detail the concepts of healthy and unhealthy depression and offers strategies for action.

Healthy depression, according to Dr. McGrath, is defined as realistic feelings of pain, sadness, and disappointment, accompanied at times by guilt, anger, and/or anxiety that stems from a negative experience such as trauma, loss, and unfamiliar treatment. People who experience healthy depression can still function, although not as well (as a rule), as they would otherwise.

Unhealthy depression involves being unable to function in one or more areas of life, such as at work or in relationships, due to a depth of bad feelings. These bad feelings can be caused by changes in body chemistry, genetic vulnerability, and/or too many painful psychological experiences that one is unable to resolve. Such experiences include posttraumatic stress disorder, and seasonal affective disorder. Some believe that depression can be caused by a severe, long-standing infection. In Galenical medicine, depression is a deficiency of the nervous system traditionally associated with a surfeit of the melancholic humor.

You may take healthy depression as a signal that it is time to make changes and take some action in your life. While unhealthy depression will benefit from the same approach, it will first require professional help: the sooner the better. Key symptoms are misery, feeling down, an inability to concentrate, a lack of interest in the present, withdrawing from others, a silent demeanor, changes in your eating or sleeping habits, and poor digestive function with constipation. You may not recognize yourself as depressed, but your friends or partner may see the symptoms and recommend that you get help. Take their advice. Get professional help.

Experts in the mental health field suggest that anyone who experiences four or more of the following symptoms of depression for more than two weeks should seek professional help:

1. Persistent sad, anxious, or "empty" feelings,

2. Feelings of hopelessness and/or pessimism,

3. Feelings of guilt, worthlessness, and/or helplessness,

4. Loss of interest or pleasure in ordinary activities, including sex,

5. Sleep disturbances (including insomnia, early-morning waking, and/or oversleeping),

6. Eating disturbances (changes in appetite and/or weight loss or gain, more than ten pounds in one week),

7. A decrease in energy, fatigue, and/or a feeling of being "slowed down,"

8. Thoughts of suicide or death, or suicidal attempts,

9. Restlessness and irritability,

10. Difficulty concentrating, remembering, and/or making rational (or any) decisions.

Conventional Treatment of Depression

There are countless ways to tackle depression, from exercise to drugs to support groups. Often it is a combination of things—such as getting organized, learning new behaviors, and becoming more self-aware—that finally break the depression's hold.

Take the high road, or the low road, it doesn't matter. Just get out there and move, because the odds are good that if you exercise, you will see an improvement in three to five weeks. Studies are clear on the efficacy of exercise. The less active you are, the more likely you will become and stay depressed. Many studies show that all but the most severely depressed people who begin to exercise do as well as those who receive standard psychotherapy. So the prescription for today is one hour of brisk walking every day. It is also known that the endorphins secreted when you exercise increase the feeling of well-being. What if you are too bummed out to boogie? Get a family member or friend to come and drag you around the block a few times. This is a great idea if that relative or friend is also suffering from depression. You may need to be a little aggressive with your friend or family member, but he or she will thank you in the end. I cannot overstress the importance of exercise to overcoming depression.

One somewhat strange-sounding tactic is to stay up and watch the sun rise. Some studies have shown that approximately 60 percent of depressed people experience an alleviation of their symptoms when they deprive themselves of a night's sleep. The effects of sleep deprivation, however, last only until the next time they sleep. If you use sleep deprivation for more than a night or two in one week, the mood-enhancing effects may drop off significantly. This treatment is still under review.

Cultivate friends. Being able to develop and maintain intimate, supportive relations with other people is a survival skill of today. These relationships are critical to our health. Realize that it takes time and effort to build these special relationships—then get to work. Do everything and anything you can to develop the skills it takes to have quality friendships. That includes learning communication skills, improving self-esteem, and taking the time to be with people.

Tell your internal critic to *take a hike*. *Do you have a little (or big) voice in you that insists that nothing you do is right? That you are never going to get what you want?* Rather than trying to get it to go away (which it never does), change your response to it. Rather than just believing what it tells you, say to yourself, *Okay, I understand that I have an inner critic, but I don't have to listen to him!!!*

People with high self-esteem also have this critical voice, but they know how to ignore it, or at least how to respond to it as though what it is saying is not true. It's rare that other people spend as much time thinking about you as you think they do, so don't take things personally. Because someone doesn't return your phone call, you don't have to decide that he must be angry with you. That type of thinking is personalizing things. When you assume that someone else's behavior is about you, you're not being very objective. Don't just jump to the first plausible conclusion regarding what someone else does; chances are good that your idea is not related at all to the true explanation.

A true strategy for jettisoning this kind of faulty, negative thinking is to consider a variety of possibilities and look for facts. This perspective puts you in the reality of things. Avoid all-or-nothing thinking. Do you get a C on an exam and feel like a failure? Do you miss out on a promotion at work and feel like a loser? If so, then you tend to see things in black and white, with little or no gray in between. Few things in life are actually black and white. Depressed people tend to have a low tolerance for frustration and ambiguity. They tend to want immediate answers and immediate clarity. Typically, that is the way they have learned to be, and that is a contributor to their depression. Life is choices, and even the things that happen to us are rarely clear in terms of whether they are good or bad. Learning to recognize and live with life's uncertainties and ambiguities is a key strategy for avoiding and alleviating depression.

Get to know yourself better. People often get depressed when they aren't doing what they want to be doing. They may want to play, for example, but feel they must work all the time. Fortunately, everyday life gives you the opportunity to ask yourself important, self-defining questions. Who are you? What do you want out of life? What are the things that really matter to you? What things do you *need* to include in your life that are uniquely expressive of you? Make sure you build those things into your life. When a difficulty arises in my life, I've learned to ask myself the following questions: *Is this* my *problem to deal with, or am I taking on other people's problems? Whose problem is it?*

Another good idea if you're depressed is to do a medicine chest shake down. Many drugs can cause depression. The most likely culprits are high blood pressure medications, anti-arrhythmic drugs, prednisone and similar corticosteroids, glaucoma medications, and yes, sedatives such as Xanax and Valium. Oral contraceptives and some over-the-counter drugs containing antihistamines can contribute to depression, and most barbiturates are depressant drugs as well. Alcohol is also a depressant. Contrary to the belief that alcohol soothes depression, it only helps you forget it for a while—and it sure doesn't help once that benefit wears off.

Symptoms of drug-related depression may not surface right away. It could take six months to a year of being on a particular medication before this side effect appears. Discuss the problem with you doctor. It may be possible to taper off the use of the drug you are on, or change the medication all together.

Some herbalists think that depression can be caused in individuals whose peripheral circulation is sclerotic, if their high systolic pressure is lowered but not their diastolic pressure. This could lead to cerebral ischemia (too little blood reaching the head), which is associated with depression, forgetfulness, and vertigo.

By lowering the blood pressure we can decrease the amount of blood to the brain. Too little blood to the brain it cannot function properly. This causes most of the problems associated with the decrease function of the brain itself. Blood pressure must be lowered by the proper means as lowered blood pressure to the kidney also means decrease kidney function as well. So it is imperative that blood pressure be evaluated and adjusted properly. It is a complicated process, which takes a long explanation. This is it in a nut shell.

Do not feel like a failure if you go see a professional about your depression. Depression is normal. The first step toward feeling better is to know you have a problem. Going to see a therapist or psychiatrist is no worse than going to a medical doctor for a physical problem. Depression is a disease of the mind, which is part of the body too. If your doctor thinks you are depressed, he will tell you and help you get the treatment you need. Be honest with your doctor! Get an appointment and ask him or her for help. If you have resources through your healthcare plan, check them out. Your mental health is worth it.

Herbal Treatments for Depression

There are some herbs that are known to make depression worse. They include tropical periwinkle and valerian root.

However, there are a number of ways in which herbs can benefit the nervous system, from sedation to the rather simplistic result of stimulation and possible relaxation.

Perhaps the most important contribution herbal medicine can make for those who experience depression is to strengthen and feed the nervous system. In cases of shock, stress, or nervous debility, Nervine tonics feed and strengthen the tissues directly, so that there may be no need to resort to tranquilizers or other drugs to ease anxiety or depression. In many "nerve" problems, the aid of Nervine tonics can be invaluable.

Surprising as it may seem, one of the best (and certainly the most widely applicable) remedies to feed nervous tissue is oats (*Avena sativa*), which can be taken in the form of tinctures; combined as needed with relaxants, stimulants, or any other indicated remedy; or simply eaten in the form of old-fashioned porridge. (Instant oatmeal is not the same thing, however.) Porridge is also a good tool for lowering cholesterol. Oats are an antidepressant and it is a restorative nerve tonic. They can also be taken as a decoction, or as three to four milliliters of a fluid extract. Oats combines well with vervain in tinctures; add ten drops of lemon balm to the dose to enhance antidepressant actions. Of course a person needs to be cautious if allergic to gluten.

Other Nervine tonics that have a relaxing effect include damiana (*Turnera diffusa*), skullcap, vervain, wood betony, and lavender. The skullcap and lavender mentioned above are particularly effective, particularly for problems related to stress.

Borage (*Borago officinalis*) is a restorative for the adrenal cortex and it is supposed to ease depression. Take ten milliliters of juice three times a day. It is best to not combine use of borage with other treatments. Basil (*Ocimum basilicum*) is also known to be spiritually uplifting, especially effective for the lower chakras; it is known to be useful to encourage earthing or groundedness. Eat fresh herb leaves, or add five drops of essential oil to bath water, or mix one milliliter in twenty milliliters of carrier oil for massage. Take up to three milliliters tincture three times a day or take as an infusion. Combine leaves with lemon balm or rose petals in an infusion, and add a few drops of geranium or rose oil to massage oil to increase uplifting effects. (If you're pregnant, it's best to avoid the oil, however.)

Damiana, which I mentioned above, is a stimulant Nervine. It's good for the male hormonal system and is an antidepressant. Take up to two and one-half milliliters tincture three times a day, or add twenty grams of herb to five hundred milliliters for an infusion. Combine with oats for general depression; if anxiety is a problem, combine with skullcap or wood betony using equal amounts of tincture, up to a total of five milliliters per dose.

The clinical female formula below is a good antidepressant as well.

3 parts lady slipper

2 parts raspberry

1 part ginger root.

Infuse one ounce of the mixture in one pint of boiling water and administer one cup every hour. If more stimulation is needed then capsicum (cayenne) can be added. For depression, one to two glasses a day would be enough to help.

Siberian ginseng is good for both men and women alike. It can be taken for extended periods of time. It is a superlative "adaptogen," imparting resistance to a large range of physical, chemical, and biological stresses. It improves appetite, sleep, and reflex action, and is beneficial in many nervous disorders, such as chronic irritability, depression, nervous exhaustion, hypochondria, and menopausal neurosis. Siberian ginseng develops the memory, endowing it with a healthy retentiveness. The Russians are so convinced of its benefits that they have issued it to Olympic contenders and the aging senior officers in the Russian army.

Chapter 18:
Chronic Fatigue Syndrome

If the flu makes you feel as though you have been hit by a car, then chronic fatigue syndrome (CFS) is like getting socked by the entire GM assembly line. Flu-like symptoms are typical of CFS; you experience a low-grade fever, sore throat, assorted aches and pains, and the kind of "dead-on-your-feet" fatigue that makes a slug look industrious. Unlike the flu, this so-called yuppie flu just won't go away—not in days, weeks, or even months. It is sometimes so bad people can't get out of bed, yet alone hold a job.

Formerly called Epstein-Barr virus syndrome, doctors are not 100 percent sure what causes CFS, nor do they agree on how to treat it. Some consider CFS a sleep disorder, since its victims often sleep twice as much as other people, yet still feel fatigued. Some think that it results from stress, since CFS often strikes young high-achievers who lead stressful lives but otherwise are in good health. And researchers wonder why 80 percent of CFS patients are women, most of them between the ages of twenty-five and forty-five. The diagnosis of this illness is based on clinical observations with symptoms of persistent or relapsing fatigue combined with at least a 50 percent reduction of activity level for at least six months.

Conventional Treatment of Chronic Fatigue Syndrome

While the search for some concrete answers continues, here are some of the things doctors say you should do if you are diagnosed with CFS.

Try to stay active. Some experts heartily encourage CFS patients to exercise each day. It is important to stay active, even if a fifty-yard walk up and down the block is all you can comfortably do. The exercise will increase the production of endorphins, which are the hormones in the body associated with feelings of happiness and that help to prevent us from going into a depression.

Some doctors believe that exercise plays an important role in preventing CFS. It has been documented that people who were active before they contracted CFS did not get as sick from the illness as those who did not exercise previously. The active patients also rebounded more quickly.

Don't overexert yourself. While exercise is important, you don't want to exercise to the point you will wind up in bed for a week afterward because you pushed yourself too hard. Most doctors advise CFS patients to exercise until they start to perspire. Then quit.

Another way to combat chronic fatigue syndrome is to get mucho magnesium. Some doctors and researchers have concluded that CFS sufferers may have abnormally low levels of magnesium. Good food sources of magnesium include dark green leafy vegetables, peas, nuts, and whole grains such as brown rice and soybeans.

Junk the junk food diet. Another thing doctors have noticed is that many of CFS sufferers eat way too much sugar, white flour, and processed foods. They recommend that these patients stick to home-cooked foods with plenty of fresh vegetables. Several vitamins and minerals that may be missing from processed foods can benefit CFS patients. Be sure to take multivitamins, even if you are eating a fairly good diet. (Your body just gets rid of the excess vitamins and minerals it does not need.)

If you suffer from CFS, you should pay special attention to allergies, as they can be very pronounced since the immune system is activated to fight whatever is causing this illness. If you know you are allergic to something, be careful to avoid it. Avoid drinking red wine or eating aged cheeses since these foods can trigger migraine-like headaches in CFS patients.

Have a good healthy sleep. CFS patients have a greater need for sleep, and while they may sleep a lot, it is not always restful. You will not get better if you do not sleep well. Some tips to sleep well include:

1. Take a whiff of lavender. It is an excellent relaxant. You can purchase this essence oil at most health-food stores, or herbal shops.

2. Switch to linen sheets. It is thought that linen sheets feel better against the skin and disperse body heat better than other fabrics.

3. Get an electric blanket, and set it so it goes off after you go to sleep.

4. Say no to the nightcap. Alcohol does help people get to sleep, but its sleep-inducing effect wears off very quickly. If you have a problem of staying asleep, alcohol will not help you.

5. Taking a bath an hour or two before going to bed is found to increase the deep stages of sleep.

It is always helpful for CFS patients to talk it out with loved ones. It helps when family members and significant others can understand the illness. Many people with CFS feel unsupported because they can't work and their families think they are just being lazy. Many marriages and friendships have broken up over this disease. Conflict in a relationship can add to stress, and additional stress only makes the symptoms worse.

Lastly, do not try to diagnose CFS yourself. Fatigue is frequently a symptom of other conditions, such as certain cancers, diabetes, anemia, and other serious illnesses that may be treatable. These illnesses need to be ruled out by a reputable doctor before a diagnosis can be made. Learn about your illness. If you have CFS, don't be afraid to ask your doctor questions.

Practice the basics of health living. Get enough rest, and participate in a mild exercise program, even if it just a five minute walk. Don't blame yourself, find support, let your feelings be felt, live for today.

Herbal Treatments for Chronic Fatigue Syndrome

Herbs have been used for a long time to restore energy, strengthen the spirit, and tonify particular body organs. Today, fashionable Eastern tonics such as ginseng and dang gui are more popular than traditional

Western tonics such as rosemary and sage. Tonic herbs can be helpful in numerous ways: as boosting energy qi; nourishing blood or body fluids; balancing the humors of Ayurvedic medicine; strengthening immunity; or stimulating jing (the "vital essence"), which, according to Chinese medicine, is stored in the kidneys and is the source of our creative and reproductive energies. Tonic herbs are used to strengthen the spirit; the Taoists use herbs such as ling zhi and he shou wu to increase mental acuity, while in India amalki and shatavari play a similar role. It is important to remember that tonic herbs should not be used during acute illness without professional guidance.

In the East, illness is often defined in terms of energy deficiency—either yin or yang—and is treated with a variety of energy or qi tonics. A deficiency can lead to stagnation and symptoms of stagnant qi can include gastric fullness, chest pain, or headache. Herbs to help "move energy," such as Chen pi or ginger, are often added to the tonic mixture. Energy tonics can be useful in exhaustion or convalescence, such as after influenza. Symptoms of yang deficiency include frequent colds or infection, fatigue, fluid retention, coldness and pallor, puffy tongue, and a slow, tired pulse. Symptoms of yin deficiency include feverishness and night sweats, debility following a long illness, a red shiny tongue and a fast pulse.

A correct diagnosis is important because the use of inappropriate tonic remedies—such as yang tonic when yang energies are already in excess—can make the condition worse. Seek professional help for severe persistent problems.

One of the Chinese herbs you might want to try for chronic fatigue syndrome is Ling Zhi (*Ganoderma Lucidium*). It is an immune stimulant, Nervine, it strengthens the spirit, it is a heart tonic, and it is an antibacterial, anti-allergenic, anti-inflammatory, and anti-tussive heart tonic. It is a herb used by the Taoist and is said to increase awareness, determination, and longevity. You take a tincture or up to 600 mg. powder in a capsule a day. Can be combined with shitake, or used alone.

Siberian ginseng (*Eleutherococcus senticosus*) is another herb to try to combat CFS. Use the root. It is an antispasmodic and antirheumatic herb and it increases stamina and the ability to cope with stress. It is less heating or heat stimulating than Asian ginseng and is suitable for those who find Korean ginseng too stimulating. Take a tincture or five hundred milligrams to two grams in capsules or tablet form.

Panax ginseng is an energy stimulant with a tonic effect on all body organs, especially the lungs and spleen; it is also a demulcent. Take a decoction or tincture, or take five hundred milligrams to four grams powdered root in capsule a day. Use as a general tonic for three to four weeks in the fall to strengthen the body for winter. This herb can be combined with hung qi for fatigue or ginger for asthma and chronic coughs. Caution: avoid high doses or prolonged use in pregnancy and hypertension.

The reishi mushroom (also known as ling zhi) is a semi-rare species harvested in the rain forest of the northwest coastal states and British Columbia. As with all varieties of mushroom, experienced identification is essential, as is knowledge of the exact stage of maturity for harvesting. Consumption of the mushroom in the raw state is not recommended. The freshly picked mushrooms are carefully examined and selected for purity; any contaminated ones are discarded. The fruit is dried as an adaptogen, helping the body cope with stress from infectious diseases and physical causes. The mushroom also serves as an adaptogen, Nervine, and a relaxant, an anti-allergenic, hypoglycemic, alterative, antitumor, antiviral, and immune tonic. It works on the central nervous system to relax a person, making it useful in insomnia. This herb has been considered a longevity tonic, probably due to its antioxidant effect. In several countries this herb is used to treat cancer, AIDS, and chronic fatigue patients. This herb is also known to detoxify the liver. The reishi mushroom is not used completely alone for long periods of time and should be taken with other supplements. Vitamin C and ginger are particularly good companions. A formula that has been known to work is:

1 part reishi solid extract

5 parts echinacea root

3 parts ginger root

1 part barberry root.

Ground powders and encapsulate into 00 capsules.[7] Take two to three capsules per day. Another companion for reishi mushrooms is shitake. Wild reishi mushrooms are one of the richest sources of true

---

7   See appendix 3

organic geranium, an antioxidant known to promote good health. Chemical analyses confirm their high content of minerals, including calcium, potassium, and magnesium, as well as a very low sodium level. One reason why these mushrooms are recognized as an energy booster is their high protein level. The name ling zhi, used in China, means "the mushroom of immortality." The Chinese use the mushroom to preserve one's youth. It is said to increase awareness, determination, and longevity. No toxic effects have been observed even at three hundred times the recommended therapeutic dose. You take a tincture or up to six hundred milligrams of powder in a capsule a day.

When initially starting a treatment of reishi, occasionally dizziness, sore bones, irritated skin, mild diarrhea, or constipation may be experienced. These conditions are signs of the cleansing of toxins from the body. Once the toxins have been removed, these conditions will disappear.

Scots pine has a stimulating action that gives the herb a role in the internal treatment of rheumatism and arthritis. There is a tradition of adding a preparation of the twigs to the bath water to ease fatigue. It is used to treat nervous debility and sleeplessness, as well as aiding in the healing of cuts and soothing skin irritations. For the bath, leave three handfuls of the twigs to stand in seven hundred fifty milliliters of water for half an hour, then bring to a boil, simmer for ten minutes, strain, and add to the hot bath.

Another herb worth mentioning is rosemary (*rosmarinus officinalis*). Used in an infusion, it is good for fatigue and headaches.

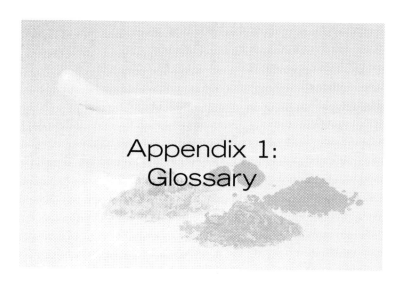

Appendix 1: Glossary

Adaptogen In order to be considered an adaptogen, an herb must have three traits. It must be nontoxic to the user, at least in any reasonable amount. It must also generate a nonspecific response, meaning that it does not target a specific region of the body, but rather benefits the body as a whole. In addition, adaptogen must help to create a state of balance or normalization in the patient, restoring the natural <u>Homeostasis</u> of his or her body. In addition to helping your body adapt to stress, adaptogens also appear to be good for you; many of them are high in <u>antioxidants</u>, for example.

There are no toxic effects of this ingredient and high intake is well tolerated. Adaptogens are not banned by any international sports body. They prevent imbalances in the endocrine, hormonal, and immune system. They increase the body's resistance to stress biologically, emotionally, and physical. They are known to increase metabolism and contain many antioxidants

Alanine is a naturally occurring, nonessential amino acid. It is nonessential in the fact that a "healthy body" is able to manufacture its own supply. It helps convert the simple sugar glucose into energy and eliminate toxins from the liver. It plays a key role in maintaining glucose levels and thus energy supplies in the body. The body must have Alanine to process the B vitamins necessary for good health. Good sources of Alanine are avocado, poultry, eggs, and dairy products. Taking any one amino acid could upset the nitrogen balance in the body and make it harder for the liver and kidneys to eliminate waste.

Allopathic A conventional practice of herbal medicine since the eighteenth century.

Alteratives Cleaners of the blood system, tonics for the blood, gradually alter and correct impure blood conditions. Modify nutrition, clean lymphatic glands, and overcome morbid process. They aid in the balancing electrolytes and hormones. They cleanse the blood by acting on the liver and spleen. They act on the lymphatic system in an eliminative way. They act on the endocrine glands to balance the body chemistry. They contain antioxidants that have a "normalizing effect" on the body. They prevent imbalances by toning multiple biological functions at once, as they increase the body's resistance to stress and trauma.

Amenorrhea is absence of the menses (menstruation), primary amenorrhea refers to the absence of the onset of menstruation at puberty. Secondary is when the menses has started then ceases. This can be caused by ill health or emotional shock; the most common cause is a disturbance of the endocrine glands.

Anodyne A medicine that relieves pain.

Astringents They are herbal agents that draw together soft organic tissue. They are used to strengthen and contract a relaxed or weakened condition of muscle fiber and to treat diarrhea and hemorrhoids. They precipitate proteins from the surface of cells or mucus membranes, producing a protective coating.

Autonomic Balance Refers to the autonomic nervous system, the branch that works without conscious control. It governs the glands, cardiac muscle, and the smooth muscles such as those of the digestive system, the respiratory system, and the skin. .

Ayurvedic medicine Ayurvedic medicine is a system of traditional medicine native to India, and practiced in other parts of the world as a form of alternative medicine. Over the centuries practitioners of Ayurvedic have developed a number of medicinal preparations and surgical procedures for the treatment of various ailments and diseases. In Western medicine it is used to complement, rather than replace, the treatment regime and relationship that exists between a patient and their existing physician. This type of medicine stresses the use of plant-based medicines and treatments. Ayurvedic medicine is said to have a long history dating back to second millennium BC. It then has some of the oldest organized systems of medicine. In 2009, the United States of America National Center for Complementary and Alternative Medicine (NCCAM) of the National Institutes of Health expended $1.2 million of its $123 million annual budget on Ayurvedic medicine-related research.

Carminative An herb that relieves flatulence, digestive colic, and gastric distention. Usually contains volatile oils that excite peristalsis.

Cathartic it is an herb that has a laxative action. They not only accelerate the evacuation process from the liver, gall ducts, and bowels, they heal and cleanse while they do so, strengthening and toning the colon.

Chakra It is a mixture of physical energy present in every cell of the body and the spiritual energy gained from exercise and experience. It is one of the seven centers of spiritual energy in the human body, which looks like spinning wheels according to Yoga philosophy. They allow energy to flow from one part of the body to another. As with all things in our reality they are linked to sound, light, and color. To heal is to bring the chakras into alignment and balance.

Compound An herbal formula. It is a preparation made up of two or more herbal agents that are organically compatible. Some of the ingredients contained in one may negate the value of the other, and vice versa. So it is important to know your herbs.

Decoction A water solution of plant extracts. They are prepared at a boiling temperature. Decoctions differ from infusions in that course and brittle structures are the base as in the roots or bark. They are usually intended for immediate use. It is stated by some authorities that they should not be kept for longer than six to eight hours after mixing. The ground plant should be placed into a vessel that has a lid. Never use aluminum or iron cookware. Stainless steel or Pyrex is okay. One quart of cold water should be added. Mix then place vessel over heat and bring to a boil. Simmer for fifteen minutes, remove from heat, and cool to about body temperature. Pour the decoction into a jar through a suitable strainer. You will end up with shortly less than one quart of fluid.

Demulcent An agent that sooths and allays irritation of mucous membranes. They usually have greasy properties. They coat, shield, lubricate, and sooth the inflamed membrane surface. Often used as carriers for other medicinal herbs. In poultices, they retain warmth and moisture while absorbing the pus discharge from the skin.

Dysmenorrhea Is just painful menstruation due to a variety of causes; it can be congestive, essential, inflammatory, membranous, or obstructive. It may not be in the uterus itself. It may be in the fallopian tubes.

Dyspepsia Impairment of the power or function of digestion; usually applied to epigastric discomfort after meals.

Electrolytes Refers to the ions in the body, i.e., sodium, potassium, calcium, and magnesium. These ions are essential for acid-base balance in the body, integral in the clotting mechanism of the blood, and are essential in chemical changes necessary for normal body functions.

Embryo A new organism in the earliest stage of development; the human young from the time of fertilization of the ovum until the beginning of the third month. After the second month the unborn baby is usually referred to as the fetus.

Emmenagogues Herbs that promote menstrual flow and discharge. Regulate menstruation to normal minimum instead of excessive or lacking.

Eyebright An attractive weed that grows in fields and meadow areas of most temperate climate regions of the world. Eyebright is a parasitic plant that must attach its roots to the roots of other plants in order to survive. High demand and harvesting of this herb has made eyebright an endangered species in some regions of the world.

Nearly all of the eyebright sold on the market is produced in Europe. It produces violet-like, white, light red, or purple flowers, often with purple lines or yellow dots on them. Eyebright has also been used as an eye wash for treating a number of different eye conditions. The chemical substance, tannins, that is produced by eyebright has been used to reduce eye inflammation as well as to create a protective covering over the surface of the eye.

Extracts Are prepared by boiling an herbal agent in water and then evaporating the strained decoction to a desired concentration. This yields a more concentrated herbal remedy.

Galenical medicine Hippocrates may be the father of medicine, but for centuries, medieval Europe followed the teachings of Galen, a second century physician, who wrote extensively about the body's four "humors"—blood, phlegm, black bile, and yellow bile—and classified herbs by their essential qualities: hot or cold, dry or damp. These theories were later expanded by the seventh-century Arabian doctors. This medicine is practiced today in the Muslim world and India.

Glutamic acid A crystalline nonessential amino acid, widely distributed in proteins.

Glycine A nonessential amino acid occurring with proteins. It has been synthesized and is used as a gastric antacid and dietary supplement, also called amino acetic acid and glycocoll. It is essential to maintaining healthy central nervous and digestive system. It has only recently been shown to provide protection via antioxidants from some types of cancer. Almost 1/3 of collagen, which keeps the skin and connective tissue firm and flexible, is composed of glycine. Without glycine the body would not be able to repair damaged tissue and would never heal. It helps regulate blood sugar levels by supplying the body with glucose needed for energy. It is useful for treating symptoms characterized with low energy and fatigue. It is used in a number of gastric antacids as it helps regulate the making of bile acid used to digest fats. It is necessary for a healthy normal functioning of the nervous system. It is then used in treatment of seizure activity, hyperactivity, bipolar depression, and management of schizophrenia.

Dietary sources of glycine are fish, meat, beans, milk, and cheese. It is also found in capsule form. There has been no known toxic effect of glycine. People with kidney or liver disease should not consume glycine or other amino acids without consulting their doctor. Taking any one amino acid supplement can cause a build-up of nitrogen or ammonia in the body, which makes the liver and kidneys work harder to remove waste. It can also increase the effects of some medication so it is important to consult your doctor before taking any supplements.

Hyperemisis gravaderim is the feeling of or actual vomiting during a pregnancy. If this is to the point where it is a medical concern it is then called Hyperemisis. When it is a medical concern during pregnancy then gravaderim is added, meaning pregnancy.

Hyperplasia An abnormal increase in volume of a tissue or organ caused by the formation and growth of new normal cells.

Infusion Is prepared by steeping a herbal agent in liquid, usually water. Just like tea. Cold infusions are made the same way only cold water is used. The more delicate part of the plant is used for an infusion, e.g., the buds, leaves, or flowers.

Lightening The sensation of decreased abdominal distention caused by descent of the uterus into the pelvic cavity, two or three weeks before labor begins.

Nervine Are used for the relaxation of local areas, the body as a whole, or more of the elimination channels. They are natural substances that work to tone and strengthen the nerves. Their function is to feed, regulate, strengthen, and rehabilitate nerve cells. They can be stimulant nerviness or sedative nerviness. Use relaxing nerviness for pain from acute irritation. Pain from a sudden accumulation of blood in a congested area, need remedies that combine relaxing and stimulating properties, as for pain from gangrene, use stimulating remedies of a powerful nature, both internally and externally.

Parturient Giving birth or pertaining to birth; by extension, women in labor.

Peritoneum The membrane lining the walls of the abdominal and pelvic cavity.

Peroxidation Type of chemical reaction (oxidation) that results in the formation of peroxides in body tissues that contain high proportions of oxygen.

Phlebothrombosis The development of venous thrombi (blood clot) in the absence of associated inflammation of the vessel wall.

Postural Pertaining to posture or position. Postural hypotension is low blood pressure due to change in position or posture.

Proteinuria The presence of protease in the urine.

Root Chakra A chakra is a center or point of spiritual power and energy in the body. The root chakra is the center of all energy in the body.

Simple A single herb used on its own.

Teratogenic effects A congenital malformation or, an anatomical or structural abnormality present at birth. Congenital malformations may be caused by genetic factors or environmental insults or a combination of the two that occur during prenatal development. Most common congenital malformations demonstrate multifactor inheritance with a threshold effect and are determined by a combination of genetic and environmental factors. During the first two weeks of gestation, teratogenic agents usually kill the embryo rather than cause congenital malformations. Major malformations are more common in early embryos than in newborns; however, most severely affected embryos are spontaneously aborted during the first six to eight weeks of gestation. During organogenesis from days 15 to 60, teratogenic agents are more likely to cause major congenital malformations. There are a variety of these associated syndromes with specific teratogenic agents.

Thrombophlebitis Inflammation of the vein associated with thrombus (blood clot) formation.

Tincture Is technically a fluid extract but in this case the medicinal virtues are withdrawn into an alcohol, glycerin, or vinegar solution since water alone, for some herbs, will not retrieve some of the medicinal principles. A typical tincture is prepared by steeping one part herb in two parts of alcohol for ten to fourteen days. The resulting mixture is then strained, poured into a sealed jar, stored in a dark place, and shaken twice daily. It has been found that tinctures increase in potency during the first ten to fourteen days after mixing and then decrease slightly in strength after. A herb prepared in a tincture form will last virtually forever.

Tonics Permanently increase systemic tone by stimulating nutrition.

Tonify To move the state of tissue, to restore to normal.

Urogenital Pertaining to the urinary system and genitalia (penis and urethra).

Venous return Pertaining to the veins. The flow of blood into the heart from the peripheral blood vessels.

Appendix 2:
Tonics and Formulas

Digestive Tonic

100 mg. glutimine acid HCL
100 mg. betaine HCL
360 mg. pancreatin
80 mg. bromolin
75 mg. papain
50 mg. calcium ascorbate

Dosage: one to three capsules at mealtimes (from one to three times a day).

Stomach Tonic

2 parts meadowsweet
1 part goldenseal
1 part fennel seeds
1 part fenugreek seeds
1 part lobelia
1 part cayenne

This formula aids in the regulation of pancreatic and liver enzymes. Take as a tonic or tea.

Motherwort Formula

    1 oz. motherwort
    ½ oz. goldenseal
    1 oz. dandelion
    ½ oz. centuary
    ¼ oz. ginger root

Simmer the ingredients in three pints of water and then reduce down to one quart. Strain, take three tablespoons, three to four times daily. This formula is also good for getting rid of the blues that characterize premenstrual syndrome and is also good for PMS-related gastric and intestinal problems.

The Clinical Female Formula

    2 parts dong quai (*Angelica Sinensis*)
    1 part black cohosh (*Cimicifuga racemosa*)
    1 part blue cohosh (*Caulophyllium thalictroides*)
    1 part blessed thistle (*Cnicus benidictus*)
    1 part cramp bark (*Viburnum opulus*)

The Peppermint Formula

    1 oz. peppermint leaves (*Mentha piperita*)
    1 oz. elderflower (*Sambucus canadensis*)
    1 oz. yarrow flower (*Achillea millefolium*)

Pour two pints of boiling water over the herbs, cover tightly, and keep the mixture warm for fifteen minutes. Strain. The preparation should be consumed warm and the individual should be kept covered. Honey can be added if desired. The best way to administer this is to give one-half to one cup every thirty to forty-five minutes, until the patient perspires, and then two tablespoons every hour or two until the patient falls asleep. It must be administered warm. When the patient begins to sweat freely, the congestion will be broken and the circulation will be equalized. In the morning, sponge the entire body with equal parts of apple cider vinegar and warm water. Do one portion of the body at a time, so the patient does not get chilled. The formula is good for children as well as babies who still nurse. With youngsters you may want to add spearmint instead of peppermint and add honey, making the formula weaker and more palatable.

Clinical Respiratory Formula

1 part mullein leaf (*Verbascum thapsus*)
1 part goldenseal (*Hydrastis canadensis*)
1 part coltsfoot leaf (*Tussilago farfara*)
1 part marshmallow root (*Althea officinalis*)
1 part lobelia herb (*Lobelia inflata*)
1 part cayenne pepper (*Capsicum minimum*)

Put in a tea and drink, or combine in a capsule and take one tablespoon four times a day.

Gonad Gland Tonic

1 part bearberry
1 part couch grass
1 part echinacea
1 part horsetail
1 part hydrangea

This tea should be taken three times a day.

Appendix 3:
Capsule Explanation

Capsules are easy to make. Simply take ground herbs and insert them into soluble hard gelatin capsules. Capsules come in various sizes, 000 to 5, to permit easy swallowing. The "5" is the smallest size. The "000" is the largest. The reason to use capsules is simple: some of the herbs are very sour or taste disgusting. The second reason is convenience. No special containers or equipment is needed. Remember the effectiveness of a herb is a function of compliance and the appropriateness of the herb. Some people prefer capsules to tea as well. Some people however have difficulty swallowing capsules,

Appendix 4:
Some Essential Vitamins

Even though there are numerous minerals in the body the most abundant minerals are calcium, phosphorus, and magnesium.

Minerals needed especially are calcium and magnesium. Vitamin D is needed for the absorption of calcium. Women especially in the over forty group have a calcium deficiency, as they lose calcium in the bones as they get older. Without vitamin D and low exposure to light as in the elderly the bones undergo decalcification and become weak due to disturbances in calcium and phosphorus metabolism. Calcium is also noted to reduce PMS cramping

There are many vitamins needed in the body. There have been very few cases of overdose of any certain vitamin. As the body needs vitamins it absorbs them through the diet. There have been many people however who suffer from not having enough of a certain vitamin. There are four fat-soluble vitamins; they are A, D, E, and K. There are eleven water-soluble vitamins. Vitamins undergo no digestion. They are merely separated from the food elements in which they are found and pass into the blood stream. Absorption of the water-soluble vitamins is quite rapid, while the fat-soluble vitamins depend upon how efficiently fat absorption takes place. The ultimate source of all vitamins is the vegetable kingdom. The fat-soluble vitamins are more stable to heat than the B vitamins and are less likely to be lost in the cooking and processing of foods. Anything that interferes with fat absorption in the body will affect the absorption of the fat soluble vitamins. Vitamin A is needed for the normal growth, good vision, healthy skin, and resistance to infection. One of the early signs of vitamin A deficiency is inability of the eyes to adjust quickly to the dark after exposure to bright light. Vitamin A and D suppresses premenstrual acne and oily skin. Vitamin D is needed for the proper use of calcium and phosphorus; therefore it is essential in the formation of strong bones. Lack of vitamin D causes rickets. Vitamin E is an antioxidant, which prevents oxidation of vitamin A and polyunsaturated fatty acids. It maintains the stability of cell membranes. Vitamin K is needed for the synthesis of Prothrombin, which is needed for the clotting of blood in the body. Decrease in vitamin K can result in muscle weakness, cardiac abnormalities, and edema.

Water-soluble vitamins include vitamin C, vitamin B (1, 2, 3, 6 and 12), folacin, pantolithic acid, biotin, and choline. Vitamin B6 alleviates moods swings, fluid retention, breast tenderness, bloating, and some food cravings. Vitamin C is noted to reduce stress and allergy symptoms, as well as promoting the formation of bone and teeth, fostering growth, and improving appetite; it also raises resistance to infection, helps keep the blood vessels in healthy condition, and lastly it is a diffuser of calcium to the tissues.

The B vitamins have many functions. Mainly they are associated with the release of food energy and protein synthesis. It is also thought to be important for growth and reproduction, normal appetite, and digestion. Vitamin B6 especially is known to function as a co-enzyme for many biological functions, including the production of antibodies and fat metabolism. Vitamin B12 is necessary for normal growth and maintenance of nervous tissue, and red blood cell formation, and healthy pregnancies. Lack of Vitamin B12 causes pernicious anemia. Lack of this vitamin causes beriberi.

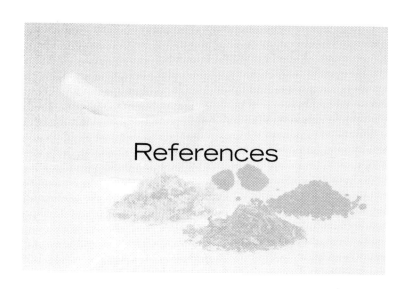

References

Berman, Audrey, Shirlee J. Snyder, Barbara Kozier and Glenora Erb. 2008. *Kozier & Erb's Fundamentals of Nursing: Concepts, Process, and Practice.* Menlo Park, Califonia: Pearson Education.

Dunne, Lavon. 1989. *Nutrition Almanac.* New York, St. Louis, San Francisco, Montreal, Toronto: McGraw-Hill Education.

Griggs, Barbara. 1997. *Green Pharmacy.* Inner Traditions.

Hoffman, David. 1991. *The New Holistic Herbal.* City of Publisher: Element Books, Ltd.

Kowalchik, Claire, and William H. Hylton, eds. 1998. *Rodale's Illustrated Encyclopedia of Herbs.* Rodale Books.

Lust, John. 2001. *The Herb Book.* New York, Toronto, London, Sydney, Auckland: Bantam Books.

McGrath, Ellen. 1994. *When Feeling Bad Is Good.* HarperCollins Publishers.

Murray, Michael. 1998. *Natural Alternatives to Over-the-Counter and Prescription Drugs.* Harper Paperbacks.

NIH Reporter, projectreporter.nih.gov/reporter_SearchResults. cfm?icde=4809741

Oby, Penelope. 1993. *The Complete Medicinal Herbal*. London WC2E 8PS: Dorling Kindersley Publishers.

Olds, Sally, B., Marica L. London, Patricia A. Ladewig, and Michele Davidson, 1980. *Obstetric Nursing*. Addison Wesley Longman Publishing.

Reader's Digest, ed. 1986. *Magic and Medicine of Plants*. Reader's Digest.

Renner, John, and the Consumer Health Information Research Institute. 1993. *The Home Remedies Handbook by the Editors of Consumer Guide and Hundreds of Leading Doctors*. Lincolnwood, IL: Louis Weber Publications Int.

Willard, Terry. 1993. *Textbook of Modern Herbology*. Calgary, Alberta: Wild Rose College of Natural Healing.

Winter, Ruth. 1997. *A Consumer's Dictionary of Medicines*. Three Rivers Press.